to Maude —
Best of luck
on your unique
and continuing
Birding
Hopefully in 2005

[illegible]

Mar 31, 2005

TOTAL BODY LIFT™ SURGERY

Reshaping the Breasts, Chest, Arms, Thighs, Hips, Back, Waist, Abdomen & Knees after Weight Loss, Aging & Pregnancies

Dennis J. Hurwitz, MD, FACS

Clinical Professor of Surgery (Plastic)
University of Pittsburgh School of Medicine

Attending Plastic Surgeon
at Magee Women's Hospital, Pittsburgh, Pennsylvania

Director of the Hurwitz Center for Plastic Surgery, P.C.

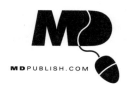

MDPUBLISH.COM

ISBN: 0-9748997-1-2

Printed in the United States of America.

Cover design by Andrew Patapis

Illustrations by Jon Coulter

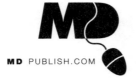

MD PUBLISH.COM   350 Fifth Avenue, Suite 7619 | New York, New York 10118

About the Author

For over 27 years, Dennis J. Hurwitz, M.D., FACS has treated thousands of individuals with cosmetic concerns, structural defects, and congenital deformities. As director of the Hurwitz Center for Plastic Surgery, he specializes in body contouring, liposuction, facelift, rhinoplasty, and cleft lip repair.

Dr. Hurwitz is a skilled Plastic Surgeon, teacher and surgical innovator. He is:

- Clinical Professor of Surgery at the University of Pittsburgh, where he has taught hundreds of surgical residents
- Certified by the American Boards of Plastic Surgery and Board of Surgery
- A member of the American Society for Aesthetic Plastic Surgery, the American Society of Plastic Surgeons, and the prestigious American Association of Plastic Surgeons
- Lectures internationally and has published over 100 articles on facelift, lipoaugmentation, body contouring, liposuction, reconstructive plastic surgery, vascular malformations, and cleft lip
- Recognized as one of America's Top Doctor's – the only plastic surgeon in Western Pennsylvania for specialist referrals listed in the 2001–2004 editions of the *Castle Connolly Guide* and *Consumer's Guide to Top Doctors*
- Featured recently in *People Magazine, USA Today, Discovery Health Cable, NBC's Inside Edition, Montel Williams Show,* WRC Washington D.C. (NBC), CNN, *Pittsburgh Post Gazette,* WTAE news, KDKA, *QED Magazine, Body Language Magazine,* WebMD Health, drkoop, TBW, *Consumer's Digest, Globe.*
- Applies the latest technology and innovations to benefit his patients, such as laser and pulsed light treatments, ultrasound assisted lipoplasty, and endoscopic brow lift

The Hurwitz Center for Plastic Surgery is located in the penthouse of the Forbes Allies Center at the entrance of the Oakland section of

Pittsburgh, Pennsylvania. This upscale remodeled suite provides comfort and privacy. We offer free valet parking.

Dr. Hurwitz partners with nearby Magee Women's Hospital to perform major procedures. This facility is a National Center of Excellence in Women's Health. Our dedicated nurses and anesthesiologists offer courteous and advanced professional care.

Dr. Hurwitz is past medical director of the University of Pittsburgh Cleft Palate Craniofacial Center. He is past president of city, state, and regional plastic surgery organizations, and the Allegheny County Medical Society. He is married to Linda for 35 years with son Jeffrey and daughter Julia. He is an avid golfer and skier.

Dennis J. Hurwitz, M. D., F.A.C.S.
Forbes Allies Center
3109 Forbes Avenue, Pittsburgh, PA 15213
www.hurwitzcenter.com
drhurwitz@hurwtizcenter.com
Phone 412- 802-6100
Fax 412-802-770

Education and Training

1963-1966	University of Maryland, College, Park, Maryland	1996 B.S., Zoology
1966-1970	University of Maryland Medical School	1970 M.D. General Surgery
1970-1972	Resident, Yale University Hospital, New Haven, CT	
1972-1975	Resident, Dartmouth Affiliated Hospitals -	General Surgery
1975-1977	Resident, Plastic Surgery University of Pittsburgh Health Center	
6/77-9/77	Fellowship, Craniofacial Surgery General Hospital of Mexico, Mexico City	Dr. Fernando Ortiz- Monasterio

Current Appointments

2000-2005	University of Pittsburgh School of Medicine	Clinical Professor of Surgery (Plastic)

| 1977-2005 | University of Pittsburgh Medical Center | Attending Surgeon |
| 1977-2005 | Children's Hospital of Pittsburgh | Attending Surgeon |

Certification and Licensure
Specialty Board Certifications
| American Board of Surgery | 1976 |
| American Board of Plastic Surgery | 1979 |

Licensure
| Medical Board of Pennsylvania, 017467E | 1976 |

Professional Organizations
American Medical Association	1970-2005
Pennsylvania Medical Society	1977-2005
Allegheny County Medical Society	1977-2005
President	1999-2000
Chairman of Board of Directors	2000-2001
Allegheny County Medical Society Foundation	1994-2000
President	1999-2000
American Society of Plastic Surgeons	1978-2005
American Cleft Palate Association	1978-2005
Ohio Valley Society for Plastic & Reconstructive Surgeons	1980-2005
President	1991-1992
Greater Pittsburgh Plastic Surgery Society	1980-2005
President	1986-1988
The Robert H. Ivy Society of Plastic and Reconstructive Surgeons	1980-2005
President	1992-1993
American College of Surgeons	1981-2005
Pittsburgh Surgical Society	1981-2005
Plastic Surgery Research Council	1983-2005
The Northeastern Society of Plastic and Reconstructive Surgery	1984-2005
American Society for Aesthetic Plastic Surgeons	1985-2005
American Association of Plastic Surgeons	1987-2005
American Society for Aesthetic Plastic Surgeons	1985-2005
American Society of Maxillofacial Surgeons	1990-2005
American Alpine Workshop in Plastic Surgery	1990-2005
Chairman	2002

Honors
Alpha Omega Alpha national honor medical society	1969
Maimonides Award from Israeli Bonds	1999
Omicron Kappa Epsilon national honor dental society, Beta chapter	2001
Castle Connolly Guide of *America's Top Doctors* editions I-IV	2001-2005
Consumer's Guide to Top Doctors	2003-2005

Over 100 Scientific Publications
The following relate to Body Contouring

1 Hurwitz, D.J., Hollins, R.J. "Reconstruction of the Abdominal Wall and Groin" *Mastery of Surgery: Plastic and Reconstructive Surgery*, Edited by Cohen, M. Little, Brown and Company. Vol II, 1349-1359, 1994.
2 Mast B., Hurwitz, D.L., "Mini-Abdominoplasty" for Operative Techniques in Plastic and Reconstructive Surgery edited by Vasconez L.O., Gardner P.M.Vol 3:February 1996
3 Hurwitz, D. J., Zewert T. "Body Contouring Surgery in the Bariatric Surgical Patient" in *Operative Techniques in Plastic Surgery and Reconstructive Surgery*, Vol 8:2,87-95, October 2002.
4 Hurwitz, D.J. Rubin J. P., Risen M., Sejjadian A., Serieka, S., Correcting the Saddlebag deformity in the Massive Weight Loss Patient, Plastic and Recon. Surg. 114:5:1313-1325, 2004.
5 Hurwitz, D. J., Single Stage Total Body Lift after massive weight loss, Annals of Plastic Surgery, 52:5;435-441 2004.
6 Song A, Rubin JP, Hurwitz D A Classification of Contour Deformities after Bariatric Weight Loss:The Pittsburgh Rating Scale Plast. Reconstr.Surg. in press 2005
7 Hurwitz, D. J., Plastic Surgery Following Weight Loss in Minimally Invasive Plastic Surgery, edited by Schauer, P and Schirmer, B., chapter submitted July 2003 and accepted for publication, Springer, Verlag., 2005.
8 Hurwitz, D.J., Golla D., Breast Reshaping after massive weight loss in New trends in reduction and mastopexy edited by Shenaq, Spear and Davidson in Seminars in Plastic Surgery 18: 2004 179-187, Theime Medical Publishers, New York.
9 Matarasso A, Aly A, Hurwitz D, Lockwood T. Panel Discussion on Body Contouring After Massive Weight Loss in the Aesthetic Surg. J. Sept.-Oct. 452-463, 2004.
10 Hurwitz D. Invited Discussion of Optimizing body contour in massive weight loss patients: the modified vertical abdomino-plasty by da Costa LF, Landecker A, Manta AM, et al in Plast. Reconstr. Surg. 114:7:1924, 2004.
11 Hurwitz D. Breast Reduction and Mastopexy After Massive Weight Loss, Chapter 88 submitted to *Surgery of the Breast*, second edition, edited by Spear S. Lippincott, Philadelphia, Pa. 2005.
12 Hurwitz D.J. Medial Thighplasty for Operative Strategies section of Aesth. Soc. Journal submitted November 2004 and accepted for March-April 2005 issue.
13 Hurwitz D.J. The L Brachioplasty: An innovative approach to correct excess tissue of the upper arm, axilla and lateral chest, submitted to Plast. Reconstr. Surg. December 2004.
14 Hurwitz D.J. Invited Discussion of Circular Belt Lipectomy: A retro-spective follow up study on complications and cosmetic result by Huizum, Roche, Hoffer in Annals of Plast. Surg. in press for 2005.

Acknowledgements

The cooperation and encouragement of the University
of Pittsburgh Medical Center and the Department of Surgery and
the division of Plastic Surgery, as well as Magee Women's
Hospital. All strive for excellence in the delivery, research, and
teaching of medicine.

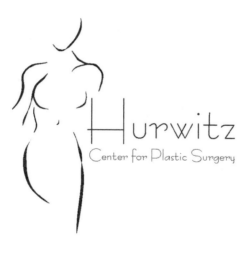

Hurwitz
Center for Plastic Surgery

To my wife of 35 years, Linda,
who is devoted to her family, to my work in
Plastic Surgery and to remembrance of the Holocaust.

To my young children, Jeffrey & Julia
who say I spend too many hours writing.

Contents

Foreword

(Author's note: After sharing a teaching seminar with him, I asked Dr. Walter Pories, the acknowledged surgeon founder of current Bariatric Surgery to write his comments about this book.)

Imagine for a moment that you are a woman who weighs 350 pounds. Only two months ago, you weighed 342 pounds and, in spite of diets and promises and tablets bought over the Internet, you gained another eight pounds. You have given up on exercise because it left you breathless; at night, your face is covered by an oxygen mask that, at least, lets you get some sleep. Three years ago you learned that you have diabetes; a year ago you were told that you needed to have your knee replaced. Your husband left right after the last pregnancy, one of three children who are now all ashamed to be seen with you. Last week you lost your job because of absenteeism and falling asleep at work.

This is not an unusual story – an epidemic of obesity has swept our land with the ferocity of an infectious disease. Over two thirds of our citizens are overweight and 23 million are morbidly obese with a body mass index (BMI) greater than 35; eight million have a BMI greater 40. These individuals are refractory to the usual measures that work well with those who are merely overweight. At best, diets, exercise, behavioral modification, and drugs produce modest, short-lived weight losses of 10 to 20 pounds, not significant in the massively obese.

The only effective treatment is surgery – and it is remarkably effective. All three of the commonly performed operations, gastric bypass, duodenal switch, and banding, produce durable weight loss and control the co-morbidities of the disease with mortality rates of one percent or less, morbidity rates of six to ten percent, and lengths of stay from two to five days. For example, the gastric bypass has been shown to produce significant durable weight loss of about 100 pounds and full remission of sleep apnea, pseudotumor cerebri, and stress incontinence. In four out of five individuals, even diabetes resolves fully, and hypertension disappears in over half.

It is a great advance. If the woman in our example undergoes a gastric bypass, her life will be immeasurably better with the loss of 125 pounds, freed from her diabetes, relieved from pulmonary failure and the nightly mask, and able to work again.

So far, so good. She is healthier and clearly better off. However, she may feel even worse about herself. She is thinner, but she is not the woman she thought she would be. Her mirror reflects a grotesque creature with massive wrinkles, sagging rolls of skin, and an apron of flab that hangs down to her knees. She cannot wear clothes that show off her weight loss; she can barely stuff her sagging abdominal skin into her underclothes. She will try an assortment of salves and exercise, but these will fail. Her skin cannot contract back to a size 10.

For two decades, some of us removed the excess skin of the abdomen with reasonably good results but were far less successful with the wings of skin that hung from the arms, the sagging pantaloons, and the unattractive breasts. All that changed with the remarkable contributions of Dr. Hurwitz who has now taught us that the body can be reshaped in its entirety and that our bariatric surgical patients can return to life with a full cup. For the morbidly obese, he has produced the second miracle.

I strongly recommend this book to anyone who deals with bariatric surgical patients not only to become familiar with the possible, but also to celebrate a great story of success.

Walter J. Pories, MD, FACS
Professor of Surgery and Biochemistry
Brody School of Medicine, East Carolina University
Past President, The American Society for Bariatric Surgery

Introduction

The topic of body contouring and body lifting is becoming increasingly popular and significant as obesity skyrockets. While various types of body-contouring procedures have been done for many, many years, the modern era really began with liposuction becoming popular in the 1980s. With the advent of liposuction, the power for reshaping the body has become more and more dramatic. This is coupled with new methods to control weight loss including the pharmacological and the surgical. Now the tools are available to reduce weight metabolically, surgically, and with liposuction. The next step in this process is now upon us. This includes tailoring skin, soft tissue, and even muscle to some extent to reshape the body into a more desirable form. Earlier techniques for this kind of surgery were inadequate to cope with the severity and complexity of the kinds of problems we see today. Beyond that, many of the previous techniques were artistically inferior to newer methods that have been developed or are being developed.

For all practical purposes, we have entered a new era of body-contouring surgery. These include more aggressive procedures to deal with excess skin and fat of the trunk, legs, arms, breasts, and face. Many of these operations are dramatically more aggressive than earlier versions and yield results that are dramatically better as well. This book by Dennis Hurwitz, an innovative and accomplished plastic surgeon, is intended to provide a helpful overview of this field for both physicians and the upper body lift. In a field that is rapidly changing, some kind of map or guidebook is necessary for patients, in particular, to make informed decisions about what operations are available, what operations are appropriate for them, and finally, where to have surgery. You will find Dr. Hurwitz eminently qualified in this new sub-specialty of body-contouring surgery.

The good news for patients is that today procedures are available to deal with a wide variety of conditions of undesirable or unattractive body shape. Using a combination of liposuction, diet, surgically assisted weight loss, and surgical body sculpting, patients can dramatically alter their appearance in ways that were unimaginable even just a few years ago.

Scott Spear, MD
Chief of Plastic Surgery
Georgetown University Hospital
President of the American Society of Plastic Surgeons

Chapter 1

Creation of Total Body Lift™ Surgery

Total Body Lift represents a paradigm shift in body-contouring surgery; an original and boldly comprehensive correction of skin sagging, demanding insight, artistry, skill, stamina, and team work. (See center fold pages 1, 2)

For over 60 years, plastic surgeons have treated skin laxity of the trunk and extremities with an à la carte selection of body contouring operations. Sagging breasts are lifted by mastopexy. Oversized arms are reduced by brachioplasty. Bulging stomachs are flattened by abdominoplasty. Thighs deformed by saddlebags are treated by lower body lifts. Drooping and flat buttocks are lifted and augmented. Loose inner thighs require a medial thighplasty. Throughout the body, bulges are reduced by liposuction. There was no organization. The extraordinary deformity caused by massive weight loss demanded a unifying approach.

I created Total Body Lift surgery to meet this challenge of extreme body contouring. Total Body Lift surgery transforms the entire body in one to two stages. Advances in surgical technique, anesthesia, and patient education converge to make this modern surgery practical. This book chronicles my pioneering effort in Total Body Lift surgery, and prepares candidates for their journey.

Since 90 percent of my patients are women, I have written this book mainly in the female gender. However, most of the issues and techniques that are described apply equally to both sexes. Men are not forgotten.

Increasingly, women seek correction of sagging and wrinkled skin following pregnancy, advancing age, or massive weight loss. Aging but healthy baby boomers and successful gastric bypass patients lead this boom. In 2003, the American Society for Aesthetic Plastic Surgery (ASPS) reported 117,688 abdominoplasties; 76,943 breast lifts; and 147,173 breast reductions by board certified plastic surgeons. Lower body lifts have increased 127 percent to nearly 11,000 procedures, upper arm lifts increased 68 percent, and buttock lifts increased 70 percent. Just for the massive weight loss patients, the ASPS reports more than 52,000 body contouring procedures. That is because massive weight loss leads to unacceptable laxity of the skin. The ASPS estimates that these procedures on post-bariatric patients will have increased 36 percent in 2004. Total Body Lift surgery is designed to help this portion of the population and is being applied to many others.

Obesity is epidemic in the United States. Over 60 percent of us are overweight and half are morbidly obese.

Obesity is epidemic in the United States. Over 60 percent of us are overweight and half are morbidly obese. Morbid obesity means overweight and suffering from related illnesses such as diabetes or hypertension. These women and men are unhappy, unhealthy, and dying prematurely. As dieting is rarely a long term solution, the obese are increasingly turning to minimally invasive gastrointestinal procedures that have recently become routinely successful and less risky. Bariatric surgery is not a cosmetic procedure. It works by reducing the size of the stomach and bypassing portions of the digestive tract. Caloric intake and absorption is reduced, resulting in weight loss.

Patients are pleased with the minimal pain and rapid recovery made possible by laparoscopic surgery. Large abdominal incisions and prolonged procedures are avoided. They are usually discharged from the hospital after several days, and return to work within weeks. They are satisfied by small portions of high protein, low fat meals. Refined sugars cause painful diarrhea and other unpleasantries. Unwanted body fat is mobilized for energy, shrinking away inches from the torso. The number of people who have had gastric bypass surgery jumped to more than 103,000 in 2003, according to the American Society for Bariatric Surgery. With this notable success, many more patients are demanding these procedures.

It was not too long ago that bariatric surgery was devastating. Weight loss surgery originated in the 1950's. The concept of gastrointestinal surgery to control obesity grew out of extensive intestinal resections for trauma, cancer or inflammatory diseases. Because patients having gut shortening procedures lost weight, surgeons electively applied such operations to treat severe obesity.

The standard short circuiting operation, bypassing more than half the small intestine, was called jejunal Ileal bypass. The incisions were foot and a half long transverse abdominal cuts through 8 inches or more of fat and then through the abdominal muscles. Retracting huge intra abdominal fatty apron and organs was very difficult and traumatic to the patient. The task of bowel recircuiting was arduous and problematic. Jejunal ileal bypass produced weight loss by reducing nutrient absorption. Patients could continue to ingest large meals. The food would be poorly digested and passed through rapidly. Patients accommodated to chronic diarrhea of large volume foul smelling fatty floating stools. Some essential nutrients were missing, which needed to be replaced. Nevertheless, vitamin deficiencies and nutritional diseases were common. Many were weak from malnourishment. The steatorrhea (fatty bowel movements) could become uncontrollable.

The procedure was too frequently accompanied intestinal leaks, bowel obstruction and failure to loose weight. Poor healing often led to deep infections, wound dehiscence, and huge incisional hernias. Occasional infections, pulmonary embolism or cardiopulmonary failure could be fatal. Ultimately, jejunal ileal intestinal bypass operation was abandoned.

From my perspective, few of those patients were physically or mentally strong enough to withstand the rigors of extensive body contouring surgery. As a young plastic surgeon, I would remove a patients' massive abdominal apron. Some months later, I brought them back to the operating room for a breast reduction or augmentation with implants. In a few cases, I would reduce their arms and thighs the next year. Through the mid 1980s to late 1990s, I treated no post-bariatric surgery patients.

In the fall of 1998, the director of obesity surgery at the University of Pittsburgh, Dr. Philip Schauer, asked me to join the bariatric team of the Center for Minimally Invasive Surgery. He envisioned the need for experienced plastic surgeons from the beginning. I was introduced to the team members including the other surgeons, surgical fellows in training, the nurse coordinator, and administrators. I spoke to packed auditoriums of successful weight loss patients who were seeking correction of their skin laxity problems. As I am writing this book, my friend Phil has left Pittsburgh to revitalize the Bariatric Center at the Cleveland Clinic. He fortunately has left a superbly experienced group of surgeons so we have not lost a beat.

Contingent to joining the UPMC bariatric team, I focused my practice on body contouring surgery. Unlike most plastic surgeons, I embraced this field as a seasoned surgeon with over 20 years of clinical practice in an academic medical center. For half of those years, I was a fulltime university medical school employee. For the other years, I managed a solo private practice, but still along side other professors. I have always been committed to training residents and publishing surgical breakthroughs. With over 100 scientific publications to my credit, and far more meeting presentations, I endeavor to share my experience with those willing to learn. In recognition of my clinical research, teaching and writing, I earned Clinical Professor of Surgery (Plastic), the highest academic ranking at the University Of Pittsburgh Medical School. My work in clinical research, teaching and writing is paramount.

I was immediately a busy clinical surgeon when I began my career as an assistant professor of surgery at Pittsburgh. I also dissected rats and rabbits in the laboratory in gigantic efforts to produce miniscule additions to our knowledge. Discipline and patience gained in those early years of experimentation have been invaluable to my subsequent clinical research. I can knowledgeably assist residents and junior faculty in their research. Periodically I have returned to the anatomy lab for vexing problems. I have re-examined the anatomy of flaps and designed new ones. Over the past decade, I have wrestled with two and three dimensional digital imagery to improve our analysis of human deformity and the outcome of plastic surgery.

Throughout my career, I commonly performed standard body contouring surgery, usually in the form of breast augmentation, breast reduction, and abdominoplasty. I did one, maybe two, lower body lifts per year. Until recently my practice was predominantly facial cosmetic surgery with a sub-specialty in cleft lip and craniofacial surgery. After a fellowship with one of the most renowned plastic surgeons of our time, Dr. Fernando Ortiz-Monasterio in Mexico City, I returned to the University of Pittsburgh and founded the Craniofacial Team in 1978. My new friend Fernando visited me in the clinic several times in the early years to help launch my career. Similarly, retired clinical professor of plastic surgery Ross Musgrave has wisely counseled me. My indebtedness to their invaluable teaching and guidance prompts my efforts to others. Fernando is a humanitarian, artist, and historian with a unique combination of clinical brilliance, innovation, and teaching generously amplified by good nature. Now in his eighth decade, Fernando continues his surgery for those afflicted by craniofacial disorders and remains a sought after speaker worldwide. Just last year we shared the lectern in the Crystal Hotel after an energetic day of skiing around St. Moritz, Switzerland.

So I started my career in craniofacial surgery, a 1970s

byproduct of the pioneering efforts of a French plastic surgeon, Paul Tessier. He invented complex and daring day long bone carpentry and soft tissue operations for facially deformed children. He teamed with a neurosurgeon and ophthalmologist for innovative radical approaches to previously intractable deformity. I was captivated by the enormity of the reconstruction, and its positive impact on previously neglected children. I had to be part of it. Then chief of plastic surgery, William L. White supported my further education and created for me the first fulltime academic position for a plastic surgeon at the University of Pittsburgh. Craniofacial surgery originated for major congenital malformations, but spun off techniques to treat trauma, tumor resection, and aging. In cosmetic surgery valuable extensions have been the coronal and endoscopic brow lifts, as well as subperiosteal mid facelifts.

After I left fulltime university practice, I retired from the craniofacial clinic directorship in 1988 to devote more of my professional time to cosmetic surgery. I left my private practice six years later for another fulltime university opportunity. This time I was recruited to start a center of excellence in aesthetic plastic surgery. While that multi-million dollar center never got past the architectural drawing boards, the move back to the university did give me the inside opportunity to collaborate with fulltime university bariatric surgeon Philip Schauer.

My prolonged tenure in craniofacial surgery begs comparison to Total Body Lift surgery. In both fields, patients have a complex, difficult to correct deformity that profoundly affects their lives. The functional and cosmetic components are intertwined, but the major issue is unacceptable aesthetics. With rare exception, a severely abnormal appearance is disabling emotionally, socially, and financially in our society. For the congenitally deformed, they know no other life. But for the post-bariatric patient there is a prior history of normalcy with the added guilt of failure. They gained the weight in the first place. They elected high-risk gastric bypass surgery perhaps against advice of loved ones. Retribution is their sheets of skin. Both groups of patients require lengthy life threatening surgery. With considerable care, risk is reduced but never eliminated. The correction in some children is exhilarating, for others there is little improvement and new problems incurred. In retrospect, I question society's unquestioning acceptance of craniofacial surgery's bold interventions for improving the sake of a child's appearance.

Craniofacial and post-bariatric contouring surgeons are artists and visionaries; creative, organized, bold, and energized.

Craniofacial and post-bariatric contouring surgeons are artists and visionaries; innovative, organized, bold, and energized. In craniofacial surgery numerous intertwined deformities requires stringing together several major operations into one lengthy session. As I complete one of many complex components of a marathon operation to embark another, I regroup and summon the intensity to resume. It is as if a new patient had just entered my operating room and I start again. Sometimes that frankly demands a respite, leaving my assistants to mundane tasks while I take care of personal needs. Likewise, the post-bariatric patient has many deformities. While they may be treated separately, for the sake of time, economy, and patient stamina, major procedures should be lumped together. Back in 1975, respected surgeon Dr. Elvin Zook of Illinois made that same plea. (Zook, EG. The Massive Weight Loss Patient, Clinics of Plastic Surgery 1975; 2:457-466.)

I have learned that some operative combinations are better together than in isolation. I believe that with experience, organization, and excellent anesthesia, most skilled plastic surgeons can comfortably offer multiple major operations during a single session.

Evolution of Current Body Contouring Surgery

Prior to the year 2000, very little was presented at scientific meetings or written in medical journals about body contouring surgery after weight loss. There were a few articles published between 1975 and 1985 subsequent to the gastrointestinal bypass procedures of the prior decade. Plastic surgical procedures were generally performed for functional reasons. Hanging, excess skin places excessive burden on the back and hip and knee joints. Heavy skin folds that rub together tend to chafe and may become infected. Removal of this excess tissue was thus considered reconstructive plastic surgery. Techniques focused on the expeditious removal of skin with cursory attention to aesthetics. Breast reshaping was considered difficult and beautiful results were rare. Wide scars with areas of skin loss were all too common. A limited lower body lift procedure has been advocated since the 1960s. Lower body lift surgery has been increasing popular since its rediscovery in the early 1990s.

With the rise in popularity and success of radical weight-loss surgery among obese persons, a new post-operative cosmetic challenge has emerged: how to remove large amounts of excess skin from the abdomen, arms, breast, thighs, face, and neck while creating pleasing contours with acceptable scaring in a reasonable period of time.

Following massive weight loss achieved by diet, exercise, gastric bypass, or gastric banding, the patient typically has significant areas of excess skin. This commonly includes excess skin of the abdomen, breasts, arms, and thighs. Plastic surgeons address these problems with many potential options, including abdominoplasty or tummy tuck, breast lift or reduction, gynecomastia reduction in males, upper arm lift, medial thigh lift, and lower body lift. These patients are also candidates for other procedures including liposuction and facelifts.

Despite considerable research, it remains unclear why, after massive weight loss, fat bulging skin does not contract down to smaller body volume. No amount of exercise or special diets will tighten it. Skin will progressively sag in characteristic as well as idiosyncratic patterns like melting wax from a burning candle. Undesirable moisture and odors lurk between overlapping skin. Flapping skin restricts mobility. Sexually specific contours and curves are virtually lost as women become androgynous and men develop breasts.

I have had a five-year odyssey in the evolution of the surgical management of excess skin following massive weight loss. Real patients whom I have treated along the way will share with you their experiences, insights, and results. With little guidance from the medical literature, I unraveled this complex deformity with its many variations and psychological impact on my patients.

Patients often presented with limited goals, such as simply removing the hanging abdominal apron to rid themselves of recurrent groin infections, not realizing that their other troublesome problems could be addressed. I soon realized that a comprehensive rather than a piecemeal approach best served most patients. I offered a laundry list of procedures, factoring in patient priority so that a tailor-made approach could be designed. Most recoiled at the large number of both the procedures offered and the operative sessions. The challenge was to treat multiple areas simultaneously. Current office and hospital personnel had to be trained and new staff hired. In essence, a team had to be fashioned. We are fortunate at Magee Women's hospital in Pittsburgh to have a talented and determined group of hospital administrators and anesthesiologists.

I was experienced in current techniques, but found inadequacies. I soon discovered that the steps of skin folds had to be obliterated leaving distracting high tension areas of pull. I introduced the law of skin laxity; whereby, the effect of skin pull diminishes the further one is from the pull. New operative design and patient expectations would have to abide the law. When a regional feature sags as a unit, the deformity is called ptosis. New techniques were designed to treat extreme sagging and ptosis of the upper arms, upper abdomen, back rolls, pancake like breasts, a distorted pubic area, and loose thighs. Once all these localized improvements were made, I could then attend to the complexity of the entire problem.

Total Body Lift surgery addresses the entire skin laxity problem of the trunk and thighs, and in the more favorable situations leaves an attractive and sensual appearance. While no portion of the body is actually suspended, the transverse removal of unwanted skin and fat is followed by tight closure, which in effect lifts the lower adjoining region. For instance, a circumferential removal of skin and fat of the lower abdomen, when combined with undermining of the thighs will result in a lift of the buttocks and thighs, referred to as a lower body lift. Removal of back rolls and loose upper abdominal skin that tightens the mid torso is called an upper body lift. Breast reshaping is integrated into the upper body lift. Together these operations constitute breakthrough Total Body Lift surgery.

In most instances the magnitude of the operation dictates that it be performed in several stages. Plastic surgeons stage procedures to decrease the medical and wound healing risks to the patients. With increased operative experience and selection of young, physically fit, and highly motivated normal weight patients, the entire Total Body Lift can be performed in a single stage. Throughout the book, I will discuss the rationale for multiple and single staging.

Consistency in Total Body Lift Surgery

The technique has evolved to the point of consistency. Nevertheless, each patient requires individualization. While the improvements are dramatic, this is major surgery that comes with serious risks and impressive scars. Most patients need additional procedures to tackle extra skin around their arms and other body parts. As with gastric bypass surgery, Total Body Lift surgery plays a critical but not complete roll in patient rehabilitation. It should urge patients to maintain a healthy lifestyle so that their new shape and size will be long lasting.

Although at times there is more detail than one cares to know, basically many patients would like the information. Many others who read this are simply very interested to get inside the head of a busy innovative plastic surgeon. For further information and reprints of some of my scientific papers please visit www.hurwitz-center.com.

Chapter 2

Obesity and Plastic Surgery

Total Body Lift surgery treats the consequences of pregnancy, aging, and massive weight loss. Total Body Lift surgery was developed on massive weight loss surgery patients. Accordingly, I start the indepth examination with a discussion of my professional interaction with obesity, and the role of liposuction. With the help of my friend Dr. Sayeed Ikramuddin, renowned bariatric surgeron from Minneapolis, I introduce his rapidly evolving field. I recently joined the semi-annual two day course on "Contemporary Bariatric Surgery" organized by Dr. Ikramuddin and his partner Henry Buchwald at the American College of Surgeon's Spring and Fall Meetings. The chapter finishes with personal vignettes of several success stories.

My recent journey into the world of bariatric surgery has led to insights and understanding of obesity. For the first 20 years of my plastic surgery practice, I reluctantly operated on overweight patients. It was not so much prejudice, of which I now embarrassingly admit, but concern by the poor results and high risk of medical and wound healing problems. The obese are plagued with significant chronic illnesses that complicate their care. They have high incidences of coronary artery disease, pulmonary disorders, metabolic syndrome, stress intolerance, and depression making them at risk for complications after major surgery. Paradoxically, their nutrition is often poor with retention of fluid and dependent edema, which delay healing. Heavy, adipose laden skin does not hold sutures well, particularly when placed under tension. The healing process is prone to wound separations and suture abscesses, leaving deep large chronic wounds. Some are trapped by their gluttony and poorly equipped to tolerate adverse outcomes.

Over my career, I commonly treated obese women for painfully oversized breasts. Despite my coaxing, most were unable to lose the weight needed to reduce operative risk and improve outcome. Their blood pressure remained too high and their resistance to infection too low. Breast reduction is the removal of excess breast and skin, transposing the nipple to a new location and reshaping the breast with local flaps. As is often the situation in plastic surgery, in the process of removing unwanted tissue, blood supply to the remaining flaps is reduced. If you add in a tight closure over bulging fat, this can be a set up for tissue loss (necrosis). Darkened patches of skin, firm nodules of dead fat, and separating incisions are`the dreadful aftermath of inadequate blood supply. For weeks later, dead malodorous tissue is debrided in the office and messy, uncomfortable dressings have to be changed several times daily. Obviously some loss of the nipple areolar complex brings great distress. Moreover, even when healing is uncomplicated, and it usually is, the sheer bulk of adipose tissues thwart a genuinely attractive result. The new breasts are broad based and project poorly. Nevertheless, most obese patient are grateful for the relief of neck and back pain and improved appearance in clothing.

Traditionally, the heavy face is even a greater impediment to successful plastic surgery. Candidates are encouraged to lose weight prior to a facelift. Important nerves and vessels are difficult to see and thick tissues make dissection tedious. The heavy tissues deep to the skin overwhelm whatever superficial improvement there is. Medical problems, recognized and occult, seem to have a way of surfacing post-operatively, particularly in the older population.

Liposuction

Liposuction would seem to be ideal for the overweight. They have too much fat, so why not just suck it out. But it turns out that traditional lipoplasty is better suited for relatively minor figure faults. First developed in Europe, lipoplasty has been available in America since the early 1980s. A long narrow metal pipe with side openings at one end and a high-pressure vacuum at the other is rapidly and forcibly drawn through the subcutaneous tissues. Fat is aspirated through the opening and withdrawn out the body with some ripping and tearing of the surrounding tissues. Until the use of preliminary infusion of solution with vasoconstrictor epinephrine, excessive bleeding would limit the extent of the procedure. Enough fluid has to be infused to cause firming of the tissue. Tumescent technique allows for removal of much greater quantities of fat than before. Larger patients can be treated safely and more effectively.

Nevertheless, few plastic surgeons advocate treating obese patients with liposuction. Large amounts of fat removal is hours of trauma to the body. Immediate post-operative care is complex due to major fluid and mineral shifts. Large amounts of retained damaged tissue may be a source for life threatening infection and drainage. Extensive damage to supporting fibrous and elastic tissue as well as blood vessels and nerves reduce the capacity for the skin to shrink down to the new volume and feel normal. Understandably the public is leery of liposuction.

Ultrasonic Assisted Lipoplasty

Ultrasonic Assisted Lipoplasty (UAL) with inline suction was introduced in America in the mid 1990s. UAL was promoted as a gentler, faster, and more effective remover of fat. I was invited to join the national teaching faculty of the Plastic Surgery Educational Foundation of the American Society of Plastic Surgeons. I learned the technique, practiced it, and taught it to plastic surgeons around the country. Upon direct contact, a rapidly vibrating probe selectively dissolves the fat, which was then eliminated from the body by suction. While there are many users, it never really caught on with plastic surgeons. The machine costs over $30,000 and each limited use probe costs about $800. Worse yet, the secondary byproduct of a hot probe may cause burn injury to nearby support structures, nerves, and skin. Most plastic surgeons do not feel that the marketed advantages outweigh the costs and risks. Nevertheless I remain among the advocates. Today the LySonix system (Mentor Corporation, Santa Barbara, California) is the leading machine from the mid 1990s.

I have treated many oversized arms, trunks, and thighs with UAL. There is no more reliable way to remove back rolls, love handles about the flanks, or male gynecomastia. I occasionally treat an overweight patient with ultrasonic assisted lipoplasty, removing over 6,000 cc's at a time in a 200 pound plus woman. The volume reduction is satisfying. The skin shrinkage is often impressive but not consistent. Unfortunately, the skin can sag with contour irregularities. Now there is a third generation UAL system, the Vaser® (Sound Surgical, Boulder, CO), with its gentler pulsating application, enabling better skin retraction through LipoSelectionᴹ.

Much has been written about improving health in the obese by liposuction, but at the time of this writing, the definitive study was negative. In the New England Journal of Medicine June 17, 2004 (350:2549-2557), physicians and a plastic surgeon from Washington University in St. Louis found no change in insulin action or risk factors for coronary heart disease in 15 women three months after lipoplasty of approximately 9.5 kilograms of fat from the subcutaneous tissues. This small scientific study cites conflicting reports of health improvement after massive liposuction. Clearly, when suction of bulging fat encourages an improved lifestyle with weight loss, there is an overall health benefit.

Plastic surgeon El Hassane Tazi of Morocco recently reported his ten year experience with the successful treatment of obesity by combining the Simeon diet with Surround Aspiration System UAL. I was impressed with his results. Not only did he remove remarkable amounts of fat rapidly, but the resulting skin shrinkage is excellent. To better prepare my overweight patient for plastic surgery, I have successfully started the Simeon diet in Pittsburgh.

To optimize care, I needed to better understand obesity. I wanted to learn the differences between the bariatric procedures. The successful bariatric patient wants to look like other people.

Weight Loss Surgery Primer

A plastic surgeon focuses on surface anatomy but cannot ignore the medical consequences and treatment of obesity.

Many obese individuals suffer from genetic and/or metabolic

Total number of overweight adults
Results from the 1999–2002 National Health and Nutrition Examination Survey (NHANES), indicate that an estimated 65 percent of adults in the United States are either overweight or obese.

Percentage of adult American women
Trying to lose weight at any given time: 35 to 40 percent

Percentage of adult American men trying to lose weight
At any given time: 20 to 24 percent

Number of calories a person needs
To gain a pound or burn to lose a pound: 3,500

Amount of money spent by Americans annually
On weight-reduction products and services, including diet foods, products, and programs: $117 billion

Percentage of cardiovascular disease cases related to obesity
Nearly 70 percent

Annual number of deaths
Attributable to poor diet and inactivity: 300,000

disorders. Diet, exercise, and discipline are inadequate to lose pounds and maintain a normal, healthy weight. Their appetite regulators are insufficient. They do not realize when they have eaten enough. Overeating is often the result of a disorder, not its cause. The tendency to accumulate abnormal fat is a very definite metabolic disorder, much as is, for instance, diabetes. The newest research provides irrefutable evidence that body weight is largely a function of genetics – just like height or a family propensity for cancer. These genes help regulate appetite, satiety, and metabolism. People prone to obesity seem to gain weight easily, while finding it difficult or impossible to lose it. This accounts for why their attempts at diets usually fail. Many people can lose no more than 5 to 10 percent of their natural body weight by exercising and eating wisely. Decades of diet studies have shown that more than 90 percent of people who lose weight by crash dieting gain it all back within five years.

"Obesity is a critical public health problem in our country that cause millions of Americans to suffer unnecessary health problems and die prematurely," former Health and Human Services Secretary Tommy G. Thompson said in a July 14, 2004 congressional hearing, where he announced that Medicare officials were dropping their long standing view that obesity is not an illness. Under the new policy, Medicare beneficiaries would be able to obtain coverage for treatments – such as gastric bypass surgery – if "scientific and medical evidence demonstrate their effectiveness in improving Medicare beneficiaries' health."

Obesity Stats

According to the National Center for Chronic Disease Prevention and Health Promotion (www.cdc.gov), during the past 20 years there has been a dramatic increase in obesity in the United States. In 1985 only a few states were participating in the CDC's Behavioral Risk Factor Surveillance System (BRFSS) and providing obesity data. In 1991, four states had obesity prevalence rates of 15 to 19 percent and no states had rates at or above 20 percent. In 2003, 15 states had obesity prevalence rates of 15 to 19 percent; 31 states had rates of 20 to 24 percent; and four states had rates more than 25 percent.

While a disarming appearance problem, more importantly obesity is disabling and indirectly kills 300,000 Americans every year. There is no shortage of solutions available today for people with weight problems---special diets, exercise programs, drugs, all promise the overweight person a way to lose weight and become healthy. The weight loss industry has long profited from people's desperation to lose weight. Most people struggle to lose weight and gain it back effortlessly. The problem is that these are rarely long-term solutions. For people with morbid obesity, none of them may help. Due to an increase in the number of severely obese people and advances in weight loss surgery, more people are turning to gastrointestinal bypass as a means of weight loss.

The emerging success of bariatric surgery cannot be escaped. Frustrated dieters are buoyed by well publicized outcomes of celebrities from Al Roker to Carney Wilson. Tens of thousands of ordinary Americans see gastric bypass surgery as the best solution to a very serious problem. Approximately 103,200 patients underwent gastric bypass surgery in 2003, which is eight times the number of patients in 1992. With little fanfare, the University of Pittsburgh bariatric center caseload increased 50 percent annually to over 1000 patients operated in 2003.

With all the hype over bariatric surgery, I must express some moderation. Properly performed minimally invasive bariatric surgery requires a huge hospital investment in advanced technology and specialized oversized instrumentation. Yearlong specialty fellowship training is offered, often followed by years of apprenticeship. Appropriately, complex gastrointestinal bypass procedures are among the highest paying in general surgery. The successful programs have become an economic mainstay for hospitals and clinics. With

According to the CDC, overweight and obese individuals (BMI of 25 and above) are at increased risk for physical ailments such as:

- High blood pressure, hypertension
- High blood cholesterol, lipid disorder
- Type 2 (non-insulin dependent) diabetes
- Insulin resistance, glucose intolerance
- Excess insulin
- Coronary heart disease
- Angina pectoris
- Congestive heart failure
- Stroke
- Gallstones
- Inflamed gallbladder
- Gout
- Osteoarthritis
- Obstructive sleep apnea and respiratory problems
- Some types of cancer (such as endometrial, breast, prostate, and colon)
- Complications of pregnancy such as gestational diabetes, gestational hypertension, and pre-eclampsia as well as complications in operative delivery (i.e., c-sections).
- Poor female reproductive health (such as menstrual irregularities, infertility, irregular ovulation)
- Bladder control problems (such as stress incontinence)
- Uric acid kidney stones
- Psychological disorders (such as depression, eating disorders, distorted body image, and low self-esteem)

Family history of heart disease, diabetes:
People with close relatives who have had heart disease or diabetes are more likely to develop these problems if they are obese.

Noninsulin-dependent diabetes mellitus:
Nearly 80 percent of patients with noninsulin-dependent diabetes mellitus are obese.

Gallbladder disease:
The incidence of symptomatic gallstones soars as a person's body mass index (BMI) goes beyond 29. The BMI is found by dividing a person's weight in kilograms by their height in meters squared.

Heart disease:
Nearly 70 percent of diagnosed cases of cardiovascular disease are related to obesity.

High blood pressure:
Obesity more than doubles one's chances of developing high blood pressure.

Breast and colon cancer:
Almost half of breast cancer cases are diagnosed among obese women; an estimated 42 percent of colon cancer cases are diagnosed among obese individuals.

Source: The National Institute of Diabetes and Digestive and Kidney Diseases, a branch of NIH

aggressive marketing of these operations in the media and on the Internet, it is easy for desperate patients to overlook the serious medical and psychological risks of these operations. And there is the issue of inadequately trained and inexperienced surgeons. Expanding the indications to smaller normal weight adults and obese teenagers should be limited to leaders in the field. Fortunately the new trend toward centers of excellence will obviate some of those concerns.

"I wanted to be fabulous. I wanted to wear my sister's cool, skinny jeans." – Alicia

Defining Morbid Obesity

Severe obesity is a chronic medical condition with a significant genetic component. There are specific levels of obesity, from mild to severe. Obesity is measured by body mass index (BMI). Your BMI is calculated by dividing your weight in kilograms by your height in meters squared. A BMI between 27 and 30 indicates overweight, while a BMI of 30 or above indicates obesity with possible health risks. Morbid obesity is indicated by a BMI of 40 or above. Morbid obesity can lead to a host of life-threatening health problems including hypertension, cardiac problems, diabetes, and degenerative arthritis.

BMI Resources: Check out automated BMI Calculators and other important information about The American Society of Bariatric Surgeons at www.asbs.org.

While some morbidly obese individuals are able to lose weight through dieting and exercise, studies show that the majority gains back all the weight lost over the next five years. (Journal of the

American Medical Association, March 2003.) Reluctantly, the editors of JAMA agree that bariatric surgery may be the most effective if not the only method of achieving long-term weight loss. Gastrointestinal surgery is the best option for people who cannot lose weight by traditional means or who suffer from serious obesity-related health problems. The surgery promotes weight loss by restricting food intake and, in some methods, interrupting the digestive process. As in other treatments for obesity, the best results are achieved with altering eating behaviors and regular physical activity.

People who may consider gastrointestinal surgery include those with a BMI above 40 – about 100 pounds of overweight for men and 80 pounds for women. People with a BMI between 35 and 40 who suffer from type 2 diabetes or life-threatening cardiopulmonary problems such as severe sleep apnea or obesity-related heart disease may also be candidates for surgery.

Because weight gain is relatively slow, those who become obese accept their increased size and the lifestyle restrictions this inevitably imposes. For the sake of maintaining a desirable quality of life it is best to control obesity before health complications develop. Some people find themselves stuck in a healthy cycle of weight loss and gain, the frustrations of which can make a normal weight seem unattainable.

Based on patterns of weight loss and gain there appears to be three kinds of fat. The first type is the structural fat which fills the gaps between various organs, a sort of packing material. Structural fat also performs such important functions as bedding the kidneys in soft elastic tissue, protecting the coronary arteries and keeping the skin smooth and taut. It also provides the springy cushion of hard fat under the bones of the feet, without which we would be unable to walk.

The second type of fat is a normal reserve of fuel upon which the body can freely draw when the nutritional store from the intestinal tract is insufficient to meet the demand. Such normal reserves are localized all over the body. Fat is a substance that packs the highest caloric value into the smallest space so that normal reserves of fuel for muscular activity and the maintenance of body temperature can be most economically stored in this form. Both these types of fat, structural and reserve, are normal, and even if the body stocks them to capacity this can never be called obesity.

But there is a third type of fat that is entirely abnormal. It is the accumulation of such fat, from which the overweight patient suffers. This abnormal fat is also a potential reserve of fuel, but unlike the normal reserves it is not readily available to the body in a nutritional emergency. It is, so to speak, locked away in a fixed deposit and is not kept in a current account, as are the normal reserves.

When an obese patient tries to reduce by starving himself, she will first lose her normal fat reserves. When these are exhausted she begins to burn up structural fat with supportive collagen and elastin, and only as a last resort will the body yield its abnormal reserves, though by that time the patient usually feels so weak and hungry that the diet is abandoned. It is just for this reason that obese patients complain that when they diet they lose the wrong fat. They feel famished and tired. Their faces become drawn and haggard, but their belly, hips, thighs, and upper arms remain full. The fat they have grown to detest stays on. The fat they need to cover their bones gets less and less. The skin wrinkles. They look old and miserable. That scenario is frustrating, which leads to depression and resumption of gluttony.

"One year and one day ago, I was regretting the surgery, I felt sore and miserable. Today one year later, life is a wonderful thing. I could have never imagined how losing 185 pounds would make me feel. In a very short 366 days I feel cute, sexy, energetic, sexy, sassy, spunky, sexy, confident oh and did I mention SEXY !!!" – Anonymous

" I'm not at goal but I'm sure a heck of a lot closer than I was a year ago. I'll get there, and like many others have said, if I never lose another pound, I'm happy and proud with myself, because it's been more than 15 years since I weighed 237 pounds. I'm almost out of the 200's and beware when I weigh 199 pounds...it's gonna be a praise party going on here." – Nannette

The State of Bariatric Surgery

What Is Bariatric Surgery?

Bariatric surgery alters the intestinal tract to encourage obese individuals to lose weight. Normally, as food moves along the digestive tract, digestive juices and enzymes digest and absorb calories and nutrients. After we chew and swallow our food, it moves down the esophagus to the stomach, where strong acid continues the digestive process. The stomach can hold about three pints of food at one time. When the stomach contents move to the duodenum, the first segment of the small intestine, bile, and pancreatic juice speed up digestion. Most of the iron and calcium in the foods we eat is absorbed in the duodenum. The jejunum and ileum, the remaining two segments of the nearly 20 feet of small intestine, complete the absorption of almost all calories and nutrients. The food particles that cannot be digested in the small intestine are stored in the large intestine until eliminated.

Gastrointestinal surgery for obesity alters the digestive process. One method to induce weight loss is by closing off parts of the stomach to make it a smaller pouch. Operations to reduce the size of the stomach are known as "restrictive." The most reliable procedures combine stomach restriction with a partial bypass of the small intestine. These procedures create a direct connection from the stomach to the lower segment of the

While the criteria for bariatric surgery follow NIH guidelines, each surgeon makes personal selections to separate out those to whom they are likely to do more harm than good. Weight, age, and comorbidities are key factors for screening. In general there are four criteria for selecting patients:

- Body mass index (BMI) of 35 or greater;
- Obesity-related medical, physical, or psychosocial problems;
- A history of having tried other means of weight reduction over a long period of time;
- A clear understanding of risks and their responsibilities for a good outcome

small intestine, literally bypassing portions of the digestive tract that absorb calories and nutrients. These are known as malabsorptive operations.

Before undergoing bariatric surgery, patients should be evaluated by an experienced obesity specialist and learn about the surgical options available. They should have made at least one good faith attempt to achieve weight loss by diet and exercise. A strong desire to lose weight and an awareness of the importance of lifelong medical supervision is vital to prepare for the challenges of dealing with weight loss through surgery.

The evaluation process for bariatric surgery is very extensive and thorough. The pre-operative assessment includes not only visits with the surgeon, laboratory tests, and x-rays, but also consultations with the dietitians and possibly with medical subspecialists if there are specific health considerations. The operative procedure is technically demanding and requires careful, vigilant monitoring post-operatively. Hospitalization generally includes a one to two day stay in most cases. Despite greater recognition of the efficacy, access to bariatric surgery is becoming more difficult. Some payers require a two year documented BMI of 40 or greater. Some payers have dropped coverage all together.

Minimally Invasive Surgery

The most remarkable advance in this new age of bariatric surgery is the adaptation of minimally invasive laparoscopic technology to the oversized patient. All primary procedures can be performed safely through a series of small incisions. Carbon dioxide inflation of the abdominal cavity is performed, and the bowels are maneuvered by specialized long instruments under videoscopic visualization. The procedure and recovery are far quicker than the standard large midline incision. Post-operative wound infections and hernia, which plague the open approach, are rare. For the plastic surgeon, the absence of large scars simplifies the planning of subsequent abdominoplasty. For simplicity, operative approaches are considered gastric restrictive or decreased absorption. For more information and diagrams of these procedures visit the web site of the American Society of Bariatric Surgeons, www.asbs.org.

Restrictive Operations

Restrictive operations serve only to restrict food intake and do not interfere with the normal digestive process. The surgeon isolates a small pouch at the top of the stomach where food enters from the esophagus. Initially, the pouch holds about one ounce of food. It later expands to hold two to three ounces. The outlet of the pouch into the intestines generally has a diameter of less than a half inch. This small outlet delays the emptying of food causing early fullness.

As a result of this operation, most people lose the ability to eat large amounts of food at one time. The person typically can eat only about a cup of food without discomfort or nausea. Food also has to be well chewed. Restrictive operations for obesity include adjustable gastric banding (AGB) and vertical banded gastroplasty (VBG).

Adjustable gastric banding. In this procedure, a hollow band made of silicone is placed around the stomach near its upper end, creating a small pouch and a narrow passage into the larger remainder of the stomach. The band is then inflated with a salt solution. It can be tightened or loosened over time to change the size of the passage by increasing or decreasing the amount of salt solution through an external port under the skin. With the lap band, the risks of leaks and infection are low, and there is no division or stapling of the stomach. However, weight reduction with the lap band requires more patient dietary cooperation and hence is prone to incomplete success.

Vertical banded gastroplasty. VBG has been the most common restrictive operation for weight control. Staples assist in isolating a small stomach pouch.

Restrictive operations are less effective than malabsorptive operations in achieving substantial, long-term weight loss. About 30 percent of those who undergo VBG achieve normal weight, and about 80 percent achieve some degree of weight loss. Some patients regain weight. Others are unable to adjust their eating habits and fail to lose the desired weight. Successful results depend on the patient's willingness to adopt a long-term plan of healthy eating and regular physical activity. Since patients can easily eat through gastric restrictive procedures, I usually plan body-contouring surgery at least two years after weight loss is stabilized.

Restrictive and Decreased Absorptive

Restrictive procedures combined with decreased absorptive operations are the most common gastrointestinal surgeries for weight loss. They restrict both food intake and the amount of calories and nutrients the body absorbs.

Roux-en-Y gastric bypass (RGB). This operation has become the most common and successful bypass surgery. First, a small stomach pouch is created to restrict food intake. Next, a Y-shaped section of the small intestine is attached to the pouch to allow food to bypass the lower stomach, the duodenum (the first segment of the small intestine), and the first portion of the jejunum (the second segment of the small intestine). This bypass reduces the amount of calories and nutrients the body absorbs.

Biliopancreatic diversion (BPD). In this more complicated malabsorptive procedure, portions of the stomach are removed. The small pouch that remains is connected directly to the final segment of the small intestine, completely bypassing the duodenum and the jejunum. Although this procedure successfully promotes weight loss, it is used less frequently than other types of surgery because of the high risk for nutritional deficiencies.

Duodenal switch. A variation of BPD includes a "duodenal switch," which leaves a larger portion of the stomach intact, including the pyloric valve that regulates the release of stomach contents into the small intestine. It also keeps a small part of the duodenum in the digestive pathway. This procedure is more commonly performed than the BPD but far less than the bypass or the band.

Malabsorptive operations with gastric restriction are regularly effective in reversing the health problems associated with severe obesity. These patients generally lose two thirds of their excess weight within two years. The long list of co-morbidities are corrected or at least greatly relieved. Patients feel great. Decreased operations do increase the risk for nutritional deficiencies because of duodenum and jejunum bypass, where most iron and calcium are absorbed. Menstruating women may develop anemia because not enough vitamin B12 and iron are absorbed. Decreased absorption of calcium may also bring on osteoporosis and metabolic bone disease. Patients need nutritional supplements such as iron, calcium, and vitamins A, B 12, D, E, and K.

RGB and BPD operations cause unpleasant dumping syndrome, due to rapid movement of stomach contents through the mid small intestine. Highly refined sugars and fats are most likely to cause immediate profound nausea, weakness, sweating, faintness, and diarrhea. Because the duodenal switch operation keeps the pyloric value intact, it may reduce the likelihood of dumping syndrome.

What Are the Risks of Bariatric Surgery?

Abscess	Infections
Band slippage	Nutritional deficiencies
Deep vein thrombosis	Pouch enlargement
Fistulas	Pulmonary complications
Food intolerances	Secondary surgery
Gallstones	Staples pulling loose
Gastrointestinal leaks	Vomiting
Hernia	Wound infections

Of those who have gastric bypass surgery, one-third may develop gallstones and 10 to 20 percent will require a second surgery to repair a complication, most commonly a hernia. Other complications may include the staples pulling loose so there is no longer a pouch or the opening from the pouch to the stomach becoming stretched. Though these complications can be greatly minimized with changes in technique and by performing the procedure laparoscopically. It is also possible for a leak to occur from the stomach into the abdominal cavity, which will result in peritonitis, a serious infection. In the case of the adjustable banding, the silastic band may begin to wear through the stomach wall. Persistent vomiting may occur, especially if trying to eat more than the pouch can hold. This can also cause the pouch to stretch, thus eliminating any benefit from the surgery. Complications of laparoscopic stomach stapling include abscess, leaks, fistulas, pulmonary complications, food intolerances, wound infections, band slippage, and pouch enlargement.

Secondary operations may be necessary in approximately 13 out of 100 operations. Up to 5 percent may experience severe complications, and maybe one-half percent die. Short-term results show large weight losses as well as improvement of disorders such as diabetes type 2. Weight regain sometimes occurs two years after surgery. On average, most patients lose 60 percent of excess weight after gastric bypass and 40 percent after vertical banded gastroplasty, but weight regain occurs at 18 months to two years after surgery in about 30 percent of patients.

The bariatric surgeons at the University of Pittsburgh prefer minimally invasive partial gastric partition with the Roux-en-Y bypass. Patients dramatically lose weight over eight months and then level off. After a year, many regain 20 percent of their prior weight loss. I schedule these patients for body contouring surgery when their weight is stable for four months if their size is acceptable. I prefer to do plastic surgery when they weigh their least. Gaining some weight will not adversely effect the result as much as losing, which leads to further sagging of the skin. Furthermore, if the resection is over ten pounds, they are buoyed by their additional sudden weight loss.

"Once I could shed my trailing IV and tubes, I felt like I was truly on my way. I had made it to the 'Other Side.' I knew that every pound I lost was gone forever. Finally, I had won the weight loss game." – Barbara

Before and After

"It's what enabled me to get off this self-fulfilling cycle of unhealthy eating and yo-yo dieting. Weight loss surgery is often called a tool. How well you learn to use that tool is up to you." – Jennifer

Weight loss will be rapid for three months after surgery. As the gastrointestinal anatomy adapts, patients will have to cooperate more in restricting caloric intake or the rate of weight loss diminishes. By the sixth month, there will be about seven pounds loss per month. Between 12 and 18 months, maximum weight loss is achieved. During the first year after surgery, eating and lifestyle habits need to be modified for long lasting weight loss.

The Plastic Surgery Phase

From initiation of their weight loss program, patients are aware of skin redundancy. Skin problems are discussed by the surgeons, nurses, and during support team meetings. From initiation of their weight loss program, patients are aware that if they lose considerable weight, they will probably suffer skin redundancy. Skin problems are discussed by surgeons and nurses during support team meetings. In Pittsburgh and most other places, formal referral to several plastic surgeons is generally made by the bariatric surgeon about six months after bypass surgery. Their medical condition has improved and their weight loss has leveled. Along with the referral, their office calls to alert us of unique issues. Patients are comforted by their general surgeon's continued interest.

Post bariatric patients benefit from removal of hanging lower abdominal fat and skin, called a panniculectomy. General surgeons are trained to do panniculectomy. When done after the weight loss, panniculectomy is straightforward, low risk, and satisfying. However, many bariatric surgeons cultivate a relationship with a plastic surgeon, realizing that they practice a larger repertoire of corrective procedures. These enlightened surgeons with their team of nurse coordinators encouraged patients to avail themselves to comprehensive body contouring surgery. Their support staff, some of whom underwent body contouring surgery, can share their experiences with prospective patients to minimize anxiety. Successful minimally invasive bariatric patients generally experience a brief, minimally painful, and complication free post-operative convalescence. They return to work within weeks and suffer little hunger despite food restriction. That mild course helps acceptance of the more arduous recovery from extensive plastic surgery.

In Pittsburgh, Dr. Schauer anticipated the avalanche of successful weight loss patients demanding high quality body contouring surgery. In 2003, we recruited full time academic Plastic Surgeon, J. Peter Rubin, who just finished training at Harvard. From the start, Dr. Rubin and I compared clinical approaches and collaborated on research. Together we present post bariatric surgery courses to plastic surgeons and publish peer reviewed studies. With Phil Schauer's recent departure to Cleveland, the University of Pittsburgh bariatric surgeons have effectively reorganized, pledging an unwavering commitment the role of Dr. Rubin and myself.

Throughout this book, I have scattered relevant patient remembrances and testimonials. Many of these comments are supported by before and after color photographs in the Photo Gallery. We thank my dear patients for their cooperation in this educational effort. To comply with their privacy issues, I have not specifically identified names to photos.

Maria's Story (see photo gallery)

Maria had been heavy for as long as she could remember. She knew she had to lose weight for her health, so she accepted gastric bypass surgery before getting married. According to Maria, "By August, I was down 65 to 70 pounds. By October, I was down 100 pounds." Over the first year, she had dropped 175 of her 352 pounds. She went from a size 32 dress to an eight. When I first saw her she was an attractive 5' 7" tall, 180 pound woman. "I was a pretty confident 340 pound woman, but not now," Maria said. She had a new problem – excess skin. When undressed she felt her body looked terrible, much worse than before. Her mirrored image was painfully bizarre. Her layered folds of sagging skin ruined the chance to wear newer, stylish clothes. There was so much excess skin on her upper arms that Maria would not be able to wear a sleeveless dress at her wedding. As it was, the excess skin made it difficult for Maria to get her arms into sleeves of any garment. So after some soul searching, she took out a $20,000 second home mortgage to have body re-shaping.

During the 11-hour operation I performed on Maria, I took off almost 20 pounds of skin and fat. By contrast, my average skin excision on a woman is 11 pounds. After her single stage Total Body Lift surgery, Maria was a very happy woman. However for the first several days, she was miserable. She said, "There was not a spot on my body that did not hurt." With her fiancé Greg by her side, she sailed through her recovery. Maria's crowning achievement was wearing a blue sleeveless gown at her wedding.

As her proud husband Greg says, "When you see the final picture, and you see the results that have come from all this, she will tell you herself that it was worth it." Greg than bit the bullet and had his own Roux-en-Y procedure and is rapidly losing weight over the past year, heading for a date with me.

Another one of my patients, Jennifer, truly had a life altering experience under my care. She was so pleased with the results of her surgical transformation after three operations that she took the time out to write down her thoughts, which she is generous enough to share with my readers.

Jennifer's Story (see photo gallery)

"While I was going through the loss of weight after my gastric bypass surgery I didn't think much about all the skin that may be left. Of course, I knew there was a possibility that there will be some skin – I had heard vague stories about people who had to have surgery to remove it. But that may not happen to me – I was working out (lifting weights) religiously three nights a week to keep everything tightened up as I lost weight. Even if there was some excess skin, it didn't really matter. The important thing was that I would lose a lot of weight, and I would look so much better. And I would certainly be much, much healthier. What more could I want!

"Little did I know then, that there would be massive amounts of skin that I would have to deal with at the end of the weight loss period. What I had thought would be the end of my life-long struggle with a large body that would not respond to my many attempts to change it, proved to be the beginning of a whole new, and equally restrictive, problem. Having lost 198 pounds, I found I was not as happy as I thought I would be. My face looked so old – I had jowls and what I referred to as a turkey neck. And my

stomach! It hung in a huge fold in front of me – I developed frequent rashes under it, it was so heavy, and in the summer, it made me very hot. I was wearing long pants and long-sleeved shirts all summer. I was happy only as long as my clothes covered my body. I had been looking forward to swimming at our swim club but I soon found that that would not be possible. I could just imagine the stares I would get when people saw the immense amount of flesh sagging all up and down my legs and hanging from my arms. I didn't even want my husband to see me uncovered. Was this why I went through two years of deprivation – so that I would have to go around all covered up? How disappointing! Then, too, I feared the comments from those who felt gastric bypass surgery was wrong, unhealthy, and quackery – they would have physical evidence that the current weight loss 'fad' was not what it was made out to be. I had, indeed, exchanged one awful problem for a different, and very grotesque, problem!

"It was very hard to pick which part of my body I wanted to do the most. None of it looked good – 'good' wasn't even a word that could be used in the same sentence with my body, my body looked just horrible. Imagine losing almost 200 pounds and still being so terribly ashamed. How could I ever let anyone see my body in its present state?

"When I went for my consultation, Dr. Hurwitz took many pictures – that was probably the hardest part. I was so very self-conscious about my body. I didn't even like having my husband look at me naked and here was a total stranger taking pictures of every inch of me! I got through it, and he didn't seem to be as shocked as I thought he would be. He was so nice, and I found that I could talk to him. He told me that there was a lot he could do – I could have a whole new body. If I wanted to proceed with the surgery on my stomach, we would certainly try to get insurance coverage, but he explained that I would not be satisfied with just stomach surgery. To make it look right, I would also have to have a lower body lift, which would include my legs and hips.

He didn't like to do one without the other. It just wouldn't be pleasing to the patient. When I left his office, I felt so hopeful, and I wanted so badly to have the surgery. My husband strongly encouraged me to go ahead with it...It was time for me to think of myself. He didn't think I would ever feel 'finished' without it. In a few days, with a little further encouragement, I called and set a surgery date!"

Should You Do It?

Maria, Jennifer, and many others did, and were pleased. Society accepts the important role of plastic surgery in body transformation. My advice is to spend the time to research and then follow your feelings. The experiences of others can be invaluable. We match treated patients when requested. The Internet is helpful, but can be misleading. There is no regulation of the Web and claims of success may not be substantiated. Recent meeting presentations and relevant publications by your surgeon in national scientific journals are important. I have exposed my approach and results to peer surgeons. I respond to speaking invitations worldwide. I write invited commentary on the work of others in peer reviewed journals. In the chapters that follow, read about the surgical options for weight loss patients and the amazing transformations.

Chapter 3

Skin Laxity and Lipoplasty

Total Body Lift surgery sculptures the body by excision of excess and reconstruction of what remains into pleasing contours. Except for the thinnest, lipoplasty is central to this transformation.

Adipose includes fat cells with infiltrating blood vessels, nerves and fibroelastic tissue. Not just an insulator against the cold, adipose refines body shape. Fat plays dynamic functional roles as energy source and storage, metabolic interaction with insulin, and a signaler of satiety. As opposed to children, most adult fat cells are incapable of multiplying. There are a fixed number distributed in a genetically predetermined fashion throughout the body. In other words, the number of fat cells is distributed by sex related and familial patterns of inheritance. Regardless of the function, as you gain weight these cells expand with more fat. As you lose weight, they shrink but the number and distribution remains essentially unchanged. Certain localized fatty deposits are resistant to reduction, even after dramatic weight loss toward a total ideal body weight.

Dieting and exercise cause a caloric deficit that metabolizes energy stored in your carbohydrate, fat, and protein stores. Your weight is reduced by first burning fat Types 1 and 2 and structural connective tissue. Hence, the early onset of skin sagging

---

As introduced in the last chapter, there are three kinds of fat:

- **Type 1** the structural fat between internal organs
- **Type 2** a normal reserve of fuel cell found all over the body to meet immediate high demands for energy.
  Both these types of fat, structural and reserve, do not expand to obese levels.
- **Type 3** this fat is abnormal and accumulates throughout the abdomen, hips, and thighs. It is the fat of obesity. While a potential reserve of fuel, this fat is not readily available for energy. It is the fat we hate but hardest to lose.

The most popular areas for women are:

- Abdomen
- Back
- Inner aspect of the knees
- Calves
- Neck
- Upper arms
- Hips
- Inner thighs
- Outer thighs (saddlebags)

The most popular areas for men are:

- Neck
- Breasts (gynecomastia)
- Abdomen
- Flanks (love handles)

and drawn facial appearance, well before Type 3 fat is substantially reduced. This aged facial appearance is disconcerting.

Liposuction reduces the number of fat cells to improve body shape. Future overall weigh changes are unlikely to be noticed as much in the areas that were treated as in non-treated areas. In experienced hands, liposuction is a safe, aesthetic, and reliable way to remove unsightly but relatively minor bulges from almost any area. That is why liposuction has been the most popular cosmetic surgical procedure for over two decades.

Type 3 fat deposits poorly respond to exercise and diet, making them ideal targets for liposuction. If you were only overweight in certain areas of your body, for example saddlebags, you would have to lose an excessive amount of weight in order to shrink the size of your thighs. The weight will come off everywhere including the breasts and face, and not just where you need it most. Most body areas can be suctioned for better contour and reduced volume, from the face down to the ankles.

Lipoplasty has recently been advocated as a method to reduce heavy but minimally sagging female breasts. I like this treatment, which avoids the extensive scarring of standard breast reduction, but find few good candidates. When a pound or so of fat is removed the lighter breasts rise slightly with improved nipple position. Performed through several quarter-inch long incisions, breast reduction through liposuction is the most minimally invasive approach. It is reserved for younger woman requesting small reduction in volume or in the elderly with large fatty breasts. Because their skin can retract, young women realize smaller but firmer breasts due to the removal of fat. Older woman have much more fat in their breast and gain smaller but poorly projecting breasts. There is little risk of reduced nipple sensation or reduction in lactation with liposuction only. Recovery is fast, with patients returning to most activities in over a week. Only a small proportion of women with oversized breasts are good candidates for lipoplasty only.

After lipoplasty there is a reduced body surface volume. The best results are obtained when an even amount of fat is removed and the overlying skin retracts to the smaller form. When the skin is unable to shrink, undesirable depressions, sagging, and folds occur. Plastic surgeons do not completely understand skin elasticity, much less the phenomena of skin retraction. What we do know is that skin tension is both intrinsic to the dermis and extrinsic by virtue of the supporting fascial network between the dermis and underlying muscles.

When removed from underlying supporting adipose, skin will shrink due to its organized dermal elastin and collagen fibers. With the anatomy so varied from the eyelids to the soles of the feet, it is understandable that no common explanation exists to good dermal tension. The thick skin of the back is stiff and does not contract, while excised skin of the groin shrinks to half its size. Skin elasticity, that is inherent dermal contractility, is reduced with irradiation damage (sun exposure and x-ray therapy) and aging. Under the microscope these connective tissue fibers are fragmented, thickened, decreased in number, and disorganized. Skin with stretch marks, medically referred to as striae, is inelastic. Linear depressed striae have less elastin with broken collagen and elastin fibers. Unlike normal skin, striae are unable to contract. Stretch marks most commonly occur with extensive weight gain under hormonal excess, such as the lower abdomen during pregnancy. Lipoplasty in these cases is doomed to aesthetic failure, because stretch marks and unsightly irregular skin folds are left behind.

Extrinsic skin laxity is the inability of the connective tissue between the dermis and muscular fascia to support the skin firmly in place. For some young adults with loose skin, particularly of the thighs, this deficiency is genetically pre-programmed. Lipoplasty for these unusual patients is disappointing. The skin will just hang and flap with vigorous activity. As there is a continuum between firmness and laxity, only an experienced plastic surgeon can judge how the skin will respond after lipoplasty. With aging there is an inadequate ability to repair the wear and tear of time. With no means of reversal, we have to accept its inevitability. Indirect correction through adding fatty tissues and removing excess skin with tight closures, such as in a facelift, is the best we can do.

Alleviation of contributing factors to skin laxity such as hormone deficiency is controversial. Thus is the realm of anti-aging medicine; a field of treatment I have studied, but not embraced. Due to the anticipated poor skin contractility, aesthetic liposuction on patients over 35 years of age should be conservative. I caution my patients that later broad bands of skin removal may be needed for optimal improvement.

"One year and four days post-op and I have lost 102 pounds and 66 INCHES!!! I have lost as many inches as I am tall!! I had a consult with my plastic surgeon, Dr. Dennis Hurwitz, about having a tummy tuck around to the back, arm reduction, and breast implants. I am just looking forward to the approximately 20 pounds the tucks will remove. I was kind of discouraged that I weigh 160 but then when you consider the extra skin, it's pretty good. So after the tucks I will be right where I wanted to be. People don't believe me now when they find out what I weigh; they think it's much less. I may eventually go for a thigh lift too because as summer is getting here I am finding I do not want to wear shorts because they are so jiggly! But overall I am very happy with the results and would definitely do it again in a heartbeat!" – Elisa

I am fascinated by skin laxity after massive weight loss. I believe the problem relates to negative caloric balance as an indiscriminate fire consuming all energy stores. Prolonged starvation not only depletes fat cells but also destroys elastic and collagen fibers. It is the loss of supporting this connective tissue that leads to sagging skin.

Obsessed with this mystery of recalcitrant skin laxity after weight loss, I was delighted to learn of startling breakthroughs in the treatment of oversized patients from Casablanca, Morocco. I witnessed a scientific presentation by Dr. El Hassane Tazi at the annual meeting of the American Society for Aesthetic Surgery in April 2004, in Vancouver, Canada. I have known this brilliant plastic surgeon, who trained in Montpellier, France, for over a decade. I had witnessed his extraordinary endoscopic views of liposuction, which enlightened plastic surgeons worldwide. (Tazi, E.H., An endomicroscopic comparison of various techniques and technologies of lipoplasty in Clinics of Plastic Surgery July 1999, 26:377-407). Over the past ten years he has been removing over ten liters of fat from many obese patients. He uniformly observes excellent shrinkage of the skin, a phenomenon not seen in far less fat removal in the United States. While a skilled surgeon, he rightly attributes this success not to his technique but to the application of a minimally traumatic evacuation machine called Surround Aspirating System with Ultrasonic Lipoplasty. It suctions high volumes of fat, immediately fragments it in a tiny chamber by ultrasound and then rapidly whisks it out of the body.

In June 2004 I traveled to Casablanca, probably the most cosmopolitan metropolis of North Africa, to see his extraordinary machine in action. I found it easy to use and amazingly safe. Patient recoveries were rapid and long term results outstanding. The improved result appears to be due to the specificity and effectiveness of fat removal. The gentle mechanism of the machine allowed safe superficial removal of fat to abet contraction. Dr. Tazi demonstrated the retained elasticity of the connective tissue. Numerous patients showed remarkably flattened abdomens and narrowed waists without excisional surgery. In the more severe cases, skin shrunk so much it was folded like a collapsed accordion. This technology represents a major advance in lipoplasty and body-contouring surgery, and at the time of this writing, I am trying to bring it to the United States.

Complimenting Tazi's innovative fat suction system is his recent acquisition of a proven European method of rapid weight loss that minimizes skin sagging and facial distortion. For over two years he has successfully applied the A. W. Simeon Method to over 200 obese patients. In the 1980's Simeon, a British trained internist practicing in Rome, discovered that Type 3 fat can be preferentially liberated and metabolized by its affinity to circulating human chorionic gonaditrophin (HCG) hormone. Physiologically secreted in massive amounts by pregnant women, small daily intramuscular doses of HCG are combined with a 500-calorie diet. Avoidance of consumption of Type 1 and 2 fat, as well as sparing of the vital connective tissue and vessels are the reasons for little skin sag. In fact facial skin takes on improved fullness and brilliance. With the help of my physician assistant and my nutritionist, I have initiated this program at the Hurwitz Center for Plastic Surgery pre-operatively on my overweight patients. They are routinely losing 20 to 50 pounds prior to surgery, making them better candidates.

Tazi's two clinical breakthroughs and my confirming clinical experience are further evidence that it is failure of the subcutaneous supporting tissues that leads to skin sagging after massive weight loss. Both the gentleness of SAS liposuction and the Simeon Type 3 directed weight loss preserves these critical structures and lead to better body contour.

For the vast majority of young patients with limited regional bulges, traditional lipoplasty works fine. Post-operative skin sag occurs with inherent poor skin laxity, over 35 years old, and after weight loss. With skin sag in mind, the trend in liposuction is to treat areas of the body "circumferentially," instead of removing fat deposits from selected spots. Sections like the abdomen, hips, waist, and all around the thighs, knees, and upper arms can be combined to maximize the potential for skin shrinkage. I believe that it is the regions with the least trauma from suction that assist in the overall contraction of the skin. The connective tissue of the bulging areas is so injured in the process of removing all that fat that it cannot participate in skin shrinkage. It is also clear that superficial lipoplasty, immediately under the skin, assists in skin contraction. But this approach risks devascularization of the skin which can result in skin necrosis. Therefore, many plastic surgeons are appropriately reluctant to take maximal advantage of that mechanism. Finally, partial injury to connective tissue may lead to limited scar formation with resulting shortening of collagen bundles. Skin shrinkage after UAL is thought in part to be due to this inflammatory response to treatment (high heat).

For the normal weight person, lipoplasty alone may be definitive treatment. In the overweight, it may assist in contouring operations. And in the obese it can be used for preliminary debulking. For the few large people not concerned about loose skin, it will suffice.

Who Is a Candidate for Lipoplasty?

My evaluation for liposuction, as for all body contouring surgery, begins with establishing patient's concerns and goals. Some are focused on one deformity, like saddlebags, but when questioned also dislike other areas such as heavy arms and a fatty neck. Others come in with a laundry list of fixable problems, which need to be prioritized. Some patients desire optimal improvement, no matter what the effort. Others would be satisfied with a less dramatic improvement if they could get by with the least pro- cedure and risk, and as few scars as possible. Both groups of patients are fully educated about their options so they can make an informed decision. Since liposuction avoids the extensive post- operative scarring of excisional body contouring surgery, it is understandably preferable to say a tummy tuck (abdominoplasty). If the anticipated contour results are comparable, then it is no question that liposuction is selected. Such is often the case for the lateral thighs versus thighplasty in the young, weight stable patient.

If the patient's body weight fluctuates or pregnancy is being planned, I caution about deterioration of the lipoplasty result. Weight stable patients rarely refill successfully treated bulges. Nevertheless, I believe that extensive liposuction is not a long term solution to body contour problems. Tissues that have had massive fat evacuated will progressively sag with aging. In contrast, abdominoplasty lasts for decades.

Cosmetic surgery is available for adults fortunate to be healthy. Chronic serious and/or unstable medical problems such as hyper- tension, diabetes, or organ failure disqualify most seeking improved appearance through surgery. While conceptually a simple procedure, liposuction is traumatic and opens vast intercommunicating subcutaneous tunnels. Large volumes of fluid are introduced to numb and vasoconstrict. The cardiovascular and neurological system must appropriately respond to temperature, fluid, and electrolyte shifts. An inadequate response to minor infection could lead to synergistic gangrene, threatening skin and life.

The most comprehensive prospective look at the stress of massive liposuction was recently reported by plastic surgeons at the University of Texas Southwestern (Kendel JM et al., Hemodynamics, physiology and thermoregulation in liposuction, Journal of Plastic and Reconstructive Surgery 2004:114; 503-513.). I agree with their recommendation to avoid patients with significant cardiovascular, renal, hepatic, or lung disease.

I also enquire of past surgery and mental health. Disappointing experiences from prior cosmetic procedures need to be evaluated. I separate poorly performed surgery and understandable complications from unrealistic patient expectations with an acceptable result. I am particularly leery of people with a hostile response to an unexpected course. Patients must accept that complications and aesthetic shortcomings sometimes occur despite best efforts. Revision surgery is occasionally needed. Usually it is less extensive than the original operation. Patients plagued with uncontrollable anxiety and depression poorly manage the stress of cosmetic surgery, regardless of the outcome.

Patient Screening

A general physical focusing on the head, neck, and chest will uncover most active illnesses, which need treatment prior to cosmetic surgery.

If lipoplasty appears appropriate, I visualize the operation on the patient both in the standing and reclining positions. I decide on incision placement. I anticipate the incremental changes that will be achieved by removal of 200, then 500 then perhaps 1,000 mls from

- All patients are required to note their allergies and medications, essential for safe anesthesia and post-operative care.
- All chronic illnesses need to be under control.
- Bleeding tendencies need to be explored.
- Complications from past operations are investigated, especially recurrent infections and excessive scarring.
- Low tolerance to pain and prolonged dependence on narcotic medications is worrisome.
- I consider anticoagulation for patients with a history of thrombophlebitis (blood clots in the leg veins) or pulmonary embolism (blood clots traveling to the lungs).
- Spine disorders may affect head and body positioning during anesthesia.
- A review of common complaints or symptoms, which should be addressed before surgery.
- The patient cannot have elective surgery if there is an acute ailment such as a dental abscess or asthmatic wheezing.

an area. For large volume lipoplasty I may mentally stop the operation when over 10,000 cc's of fat is evacuated. For safety's sake we complete lipoplasty on a subsequent operative session.

Subtle skin laxity is difficult to diagnose. When it is suspected, the patient is over 35 years, and a large volume of fat is to be removed, I caution about sagging. I encourage pre- and post-operative suction/massage therapy with Endermologie®. It usually reduces tissue laxity by improving the quality of the subcutaneous connective tissue and vasculature. Also I use UAL and circumferential suction. I rarely perform lipoplasty with demonstrable skin laxity. While these patients look better in clothes, most find the sagging unacceptable. The patients appreciate that follow up skin excision may be needed.

The physical exam assesses aesthetics and seeks confounding medical conditions. Under the stress of surgery minor acute medical problems may worsen. I examine the objectionable contours.

- Where are the unaesthetic bulges located?
- How excessive are each of them?
- Are the bulges out of proportion or just generalized obesity?
- To what extent are the bulges asymmetrical?
- To what extent are they due to excess subcutaneous fat, skin or fascial laxity, or intra abdominal fat?
- What is the location and quality of nearby pre-existing scars (from hernia, abdominal surgery, hysterectomy, etc.)
- What is the skin quality, texture, tone, and hydration?
- Are muscle deficiencies or hernias present?
- Is there a feminine form and can it be improved?

The Basics of Lipoplasty

Lipoplasty is technically straightforward, but artistically challenging.

The artistic use of liposuction to change body shape is called lipoplasty. Lipoplasty is technically straightforward, but aesthetically challenging. Like sculpting a lump of clay, minute adjustments in volume has cosmetic ramifications. Standard lipoplasty takes two steps. First, there is a preparatory infusion of fluid. Second, there is extraction of fat. Pre-operatively in a private room I mark the extraction pattern on my standing patient and photograph for later comparison. This is our time to plan the proposed procedure. Patients are comforted to know of this opportunity to communicate immediately prior to surgery.

I perform major lipoplasty, involving several body areas and over 1,000 cc's of fat extraction, in Magee Women's Hospital, a tertiary care hospital located near my office. This precaution has contributed to zero medical complications. After general anesthesia has been induced and antiseptic preparation completed, several quarter-inch long incisions are made near the sites where fat is to be removed. Long cannulas are used to infuse a wetting solution that induces prolonged local anesthesia, reduces bleeding, and improves fat extraction. According to the super wet technique, large volumes of saline are infiltrated about equal to the anticipated amount of fat extraction. If I plan to remove two liters of fat, I infuse about two liters of fluid. As the epinephrine takes effect, one can see broad areas of pale vasoconstricted skin.

After waiting ten minutes for the medications to take effect, I remove fat through small incisions with deliberate strokes of a cannula. I use various sizes and dimensions of cannulae, which are hollow, thin tubular instruments with holes near one end to trap the fat. The width of the cannula is no more than 4 millimeters. The cannula is attached to suction tubing connected to a high-pressure vacuum system through which the excess fat is evacuated.

For smaller volume removals, I prefer the Tulip® Syringe System (Tulip Medical, San Diego, California). I like the feel of this self-contained instrument with excellent gliding cannula. They have highly polished surfaces that slip through the fatty tissues with minimum friction or damage. The openings are blunted to prevent lacerating tissue. There is no noisy vacuum machine to break down.

Suction cannulas are inserted under the skin, moved back and forth in a criss-cross pattern to extract fat cells. I complete the procedure when the desired contour and symmetry has been achieved. The patient is monitored for fluid hydration. For removals of over 2,000 cc's of fat (equivalent to 5 pounds), patient monitoring looks early signs of medication toxicity.

Years of extensive experience and technical advances have improved my results. There are certain areas of the body to be avoided due to tight adherence to deep fascia. An example is along the outside thighs just below the saddlebags. Suction there is likely to lead to indentations or healing complications such as seroma. Seroma is a pooling of clear fluid that may have to be needle aspirated. I can better access undesirable pre-operative skin laxity and adjust technique and expectations accordingly. Pre-surgical super wet infusion of saline with xylocaine and epinephrine expedites fat removal. The epinephrine decreases the blood loss, swelling, and bruising. The xylocaine provides many hours of pain relief. For small amounts of fat, using slow and gentle care, the tumescent solution may be the only anesthetic given, or it can be supplemented with sedatives. For large volume fat removals, my physician assistant preliminarily extracts much fat. Then I complete the final contouring. This approach dramatically shortens the operation, which speeds recovery without sacrificing quality.

Lipoplasty is the fundamental operation of body contouring. Since I started practicing plastic surgery before liposuction was available in the United States, I fully appreciate the truly extraordinary procedure that it is. For small contour deformity, lipoplasty offers great results with minimal risk, scars, or down time. Liposuction is also an adjunct during excisional body contouring surgery. (See photo gallery, page 7)

Ultrasonic Assisted Lipoplasty (UAL)

Ultrasonic assisted lipoplasty dissolves fat for subsequent extraction by suction. UAL also promotes skin shrinkage. Ultrasonic waves at 27 kilo hertz emanate from a hand piece and transmit through a titanium metal rod to contact adipose. This high frequency sound energy dissolves the fat through direct percussion (hammer effect) and a process called cavitation. Cavitation is the consolidation of gaseous micro pockets that disrupt fragile fat cell membranes. The released triglycerides and emulsion are readily evacuated through standard suction.

The United States standby in ultrasonic assisted lipoplasty for the past ten years has been the LySonix System, which features inline suction to monitor the quality of the fat extraction. With care, it functions very well, but healing may be slightly prolonged due to thermal injury. Until recently I reserved ultrasonic assisted lipoplasty for large volume and fibrous areas of male breasts, upper abdomen, flanks, and back, or secondary surgery. Since the advent of LipoSelection℠ by Vaser®, UAL has become common in my practice.

The Vaser® is the third generation system that emanates less heat per effective fat dissolution. While on the Sound Surgical Technologies Scientific Advisory Board in the late 1990s, I helped design this technology, which is gaining in popularity. For my efforts I have unexercised stock options, which is a potential conflict of interest. The company founder, Bill Cimino, PhD., designed thinner solid probes with a series of grooves to diffuse power intensity while maintaining effectiveness. He also patented a pulsating pattern that reduces damaging heat. As in the LySonix system, generous pre-operative cool infiltration with epinephrine, xylocaine, and saline is essential for safety.

VASER® assisted lipoplasty liquefies fat with minimal injury to subcutaneous supporting tissues. Sound Surgical Technologies call this LipoSelection℠. My experience confirms the effectiveness of VASER® with no internal burns, seroma, or prolonged numbness. In addition, Sound Surgical Technologies integrates Precision Fluid Management System℠ for accurate fluid infiltration and small diameter VentX™ vented aspiration cannula. Because of gentleness and skin contraction potential, I apply LipoSelection℠ to most of my lipoplasty patients.

Power Assisted Lipoplasty (PAL)

Another recent technological addition to liposuction is power assisted lipoplasty. The cannula is attached to a modified electrically driven reciprocating surgical saw. Rapid back and forward motion with attached suction removes fat easier and faster than the manual systems. We have the MicroAire® PAL available at Magee Women's hospital, so I have used it upon patient request. The primary advantage is less physical exertion, making fat extraction easier. I fear that the unrestrained high force of this adapted power saw may be excessively traumatic to the connective tissue, delaying healing and skin contraction. Nevertheless, a number of well recognized lipoplasty surgeons advocate power assisted lipoplasty.

Non-Surgical Body Contouring Devices

Non-invasive body contouring is evolving. These expensive high tech applications temporarily improve mild skin laxity. I believe these modalities can also be adjuncts to the treatment of major skin contour and laxity problems and are best integrated into a treatment plan designed by plastic surgeons.

Laser lipolisis from Italy are injections targeted to fat through a fiber optic laser. Up to 500 grams of dissolved fat can be absorbed and excreted by the body. Improvement of cellulite is unpredictable. Supportive surgeons believe results are comparable to traditional small lipoplasty. SonoSculpt™ (LipoSonix) is based on high intensity external ultrasound to disrupt and reduce fat. Clinical trials are in progress. Ultrashape® is a promising Israeli process that employs a patented (US Patent #US6607498) external ultrasound waves to treat localized fat deposits. Impressive results are shown for mild to moderate contour deformity. Claim as to the safety, efficacy, and specificity (fat only) of these non-surgical devices have so far not been substantiated by clinical trials in America.

Chapter 4

Motivation, Innovation and Principles

Total Body Lift surgery is for healthy people, who accept coordinated and extensive operations to improve dramatically the appearance of their trunk and thighs. Patients should be offered a grand vision for body transformation. Total Body Lift surgery is a concept and in every case a *tour de force*. While applicable to body changes of multiple pregnancies and middle age, it is singularly relevant to the massive weight loss patient.

Patient Motivation

Within weeks of gastric bypass, the patient returns to normal activities. After months, she enjoys rapid weight loss and increased well-being. Within a year, the once obese woman metamorphoses into a healthy productive person. Yet she is embarrassed by rolls of unsightly skin. She endeavors to take true control of her lift by adopting a physically vigorous and nutritionally healthy lifestyle. These changes strain interpersonal relationships. Her partner will either adapt or be cast aside for a brighter future. Her new lease on life begs no compromise. Regretful of precious time lost to the shame of obesity, this energized woman insists on attaining optimal shape. For once, life's priorities center on her aspirations. Her redundant skin need no longer be folded under over-sized sexless garments.

For the ravages of multiple pregnancies, I modify Total Body Lift surgery.(**See photo gallery, page 32**) The lower abdominal wall is flaccid, presenting a pot belly with loose flapping skin. Stretch marks are like spots on a leopard. The inner thighs are limp. If the breasts have not flattened from years of feedings, they are at least shallow remnants of their former appearance. Having completed her biological duty to family and society, this still vibrant woman wants to restore her figure to new levels. At work, she lacks a commanding presence. She wants to wear smart fashions at the beach and the country club. She will not accept old lady swimsuits. At social gatherings she desires positive attention from her husband and friends.

Enlarging the breasts with saline filled silicone implants may not be enough. Many want improved symmetry and better shaped and positioned nipples. Breast reshaping through rearranging flaps, called mastopexy, is increasingly being requested despite additional but inconspicuous scars. Abdominoplasty has the dual roll of removing most stretch marks and loose skin as well as suture tightening of the protuberant bellies. Only the lower body lift can resolve the hated saddlebag deformity, leaving a bikini string like scar. While gaining her hoped for silhouette, this new woman maintains perspective of her biological role.

In our fast paced society, middle-aged women sometimes feel neglected or at least under appreciated. While content in their social setting, they nevertheless seek an attractive physical change. Too young to benefit from a facelift, many turn to body lift surgery. Aging skin is like skin after weight loss. I must remove sagging skin and pull tightly. The protuberant abdomen and added poundage of menopause can be sucked away in concert with a standard abdominoplasty. (See photo gallery, page 7) Inner thighs on the run no longer painfully rub together after the medial thighplasty. A supple projecting breast, the essence of youthful appearance, is the end result of a well-executed mastopexy or breast reduction.

Most seeking consultation for body contouring know of my originating role in Total Body Lift surgery. They learn through referring clinics, physicians, other patients, the Internet, or the media. They enquire about whether they are good candidates, the number and order of stages, techniques involved, risks, and the costs. The answers to these questions are individualized and based on surgical principles, personal impressions, and experience.

Like five day a week bodybuilders, candidates for Total Body Lift surgery are dedicated to the task. They take on immeasurable risk in a quest for a better life. They interrupt their life for day-long operations, weeks of pain, and months of convalescence. They justify lost wages and high costs.

"In 2001, I had the gastric bypass surgery and lost approximately 265 pounds. I met Dr. Hurwitz a year ago and have had three surgeries: the tummy tuck and lower body lift, a breast reduction and upper body lift, and then the arm reduction, all in a nine to ten month period. I have gone from a size 4X or 32 to a Medium/10-12. The surgeries have not been easy; there have been complications – swellings, infections, etc., but I would gladly do it all over again." – Dana

Innovation

I learned basic body contouring operations during my seven years of surgical training at Yale, Dartmouth, and the University of Pittsburgh. Since training I remain at the cutting edge by participating at scientific meetings and studying medical journals. I try to reconcile available knowledge with clinical experience. Understandably, there are a variety of acceptable techniques suitable for similar problems. These differences vary from subtle to contradictory. To improve my results, I followed prescribed techniques as faithfully as possible until they fail to meet my standards. Plastic surgery is the skillful application of an arsenal of operations.

When I increased my activity in body contouring surgery five years ago, I went against the trend of minimalist surgery and elected a comprehensive approach. (See Hurwitz D. Invited Discussion of Optimizing body contour in massive weight loss patients: the modified vertical abdominoplasty by da Costa LF, Landecker A, Manta AM, et al in *Plast. Reconstr. Surg.* 114:7:1924, 2004. and Hurwitz, D.J. Invited Discussion of Circular Belt Lipectomy: A retrospective follow up study on complications and cosmetic result by Huizum, Roche, Hoffer in *Annals of Plast. Surg.* in press for 2005.) During my first years of immersion in body contouring surgery, I identified recurring limitations and inefficiencies. Before I could proceed with Total Body Lift surgery, I had to correct those problems.

Furthermore, body contouring surgery is both time consuming and precise. For operations to be completed in a reasonable period of time, there must be sound planning, organization, and execution. Innovation begins with observation and continues with obsessive inquiry and self-examination. Innovation is usually incremental. With little precedent for the weight loss patient, I had the freedom to explore surgical alternatives. When I discovered techniques, I am obliged to teach them to my residents in training. I share them with fellow plastic surgeons through lectures and publications. While these innovations worked, I have to fight for acceptance. The reaction of my colleagues is informative and refines concepts.

Surgery evolves. Most advances in plastic surgery are achieved through technical innovation. Over my career I have described some original techniques, which have become for now the standard of care. I have been around long enough to see my published advances incorporated by serious surgeons worldwide, with some taking the advance a step further.

Patients with difficult and complex clinical problems understand that their case has unique issues requiring novel solutions. Plastic surgeons innovate frequently to solve difficult clinical problems. Few of us take the time and have the discipline to subject their innovations to peer scrutiny. When I acquire a new technique through others or by my own design, I inform my patients that the new way is likely to yield an improved outcome. However, until I have gained considerable experience, the results are less certain. Each new technique and technology has to stand the test of time.

Publication in scientific journals does not mean acceptance, only that the abstracts and manuscripts have been reviewed by other physician authorities for methodology, originality, clarity, and value. The basic procedures that you are about to discover are accepted, but my contributions should be considered work in progress. I have had enough personal experience to offer them to you confidently, but undoubtedly further refinements will be forthcoming.

Not Reality Television

Do not confuse Total Body Lift surgery with multiple major cosmetic operations extravagances as popularized by reality television. I do not advocate that approach. Candidates present with several disfigurements. A surgeon offers to correct those and a number of other suggested features to satisfy their concept of beauty. The surgery is typically followed by cosmetic dentistry, refractive eye surgery, hair removal in addition to lavish gowns, glamour makeup, etc. A well-produced reality drama unfolds, simulating a real world experience no one lives. While I welcome the considerable positive attention given to well-performed cosmetic surgery by experienced board certified plastic surgeons – some of whom are good friends of mine – these programs have sanitized surgery for the consumer. Viewer expectations become too high, and concerns too low. Meanwhile the American Board of Plastic Surgery reaffirmed in 2005 that free surgery on demand for contestants is an ethical violation subject to sanctions.

I aim for my body contouring patient to have specific goals, reasonable expectations, and an understanding of risk. The massive weight loss patient is not trying to improve upon normal but to correct recently acquired unacceptable deformity from neck to knees. She comes to me considering a full body aesthetic reconstruction. She prioritizes the order, but does not want to ignore anything. I combine operations for the fewest visits to the operating room.

Cosmetic surgery seeks to improve a normal condition. A facelift treats aging. While not readily accepted by some, wrinkling of the face is a normal condition. Similarly, silicone breast implant augmentation typically involves the enlargement of normal but small breasts. While the approval rating for cosmetic surgery is approaching 50 percent, there are many more who are reluctant. My experience with so many happy patients after successful cosmetic surgery makes me a confirmed advocate. While the ultimate goal of body contouring is improved aesthetics, the underlying problem is an abnormality – excess skin and fat. One needs no further justification for those who so wish to prioritize their resources and time. The techniques are reconstructive and massive. Total Body Lift surgery is remarkably similar in concept to craniofacial surgery.

Until 2003, I was Medical Director of the Cleft and Craniofacial team at the University of Pittsburgh. While not apparent at first, there are many similarities with body contouring after weight loss. Teamwork is essential for both disciplines. The goal is complex aesthetic reconstruction. I still perform a steady stream of facial cosmetic and reconstructive surgery. On three occasions in 2004, the nationally syndicated Montel Williams talk show presented my gratifying long-term treatment of three children with major congenital facial deformity. The production crew came to Pittsburgh and filmed live surgery on two complicated cases. The beautiful results achieved on three happy and successful young people were exhibited. Portions of the show can be viewed on www.hurwitzcenter.com. Currently my creative attention is being absorbed by the challenges of body contouring surgery.

Principles

Before we turn to the specific operations, I present ten essential surgical principles of successful technique. My reader should be fascinated by the logic and consistency that guides surgical decision-making. The rationale for the technique will be evident with these principles in mind.

Principles

1 **Properly analyze the patient and the deformity.** For example, be wary of upper abdominal fullness due to excessive intra abdominal girth, which cannot be treated with abdominoplasty until there is further weight loss.

2 **Efficiency.** A planned and deliberate approach avoids repetition in execution and unnecessary blood loss. Inefficiency lengthens an already long operation; thereby, increasing hemorrhage, tissue trauma, surgeon fatigue, and costs, which promote prolonged convalescence with increased risk of medical and wound healing complications. Develop a **consistent procedure** so that your assistants can anticipate your needs.

3 **Excise skin transversely.** Skin redundancy is predominantly vertical so remove broad horizontal bands of skin.

4 **Plan incisions properly.** Transverse scars can be placed within underwear and are less likely to hypertrophy.

5 **Focus on the tensions and contour left behind.** The surgeon should not be preoccupied by the magnitude of the skin excision but rather should plan on the resulting tissue tensions. In anticipation of contour depression along excessively tense long suture lines, I leave extra deep adipose tissue during the resection of skin.

6 **Gentle preservation of the incision line dermis and subcutaneous fascia.** I limit my use of tissue burning electrocautery and incise perpendicular with a scalpel. The subsequent tight closure will be more secure because of the reduced inflammation and necrotic tissue. Stitch abscesses and wound separation are less likely.

7 **Limit liposuction of flaps and keep it as gentle as possible.** That means prior generous saline infiltration of xylocaine and epinephrine, and a limited course with ultrasound probe before liposuction.

8 **High-tension two layer skin flap closure** due to the poor skin elasticity, expedited by relieving the tension during closure by preliminary approximation of skin edges with towel clips and most favorable repositioning of limbs or body.

9 **Close wounds as expeditiously as possible over long dwelling suction catheters** to reduce swelling, infection rate, phlebitis, and seroma. A secure two layer closure is optimal. Elasticized garments with minimal pressure over the lower abdomen are comfortable and reassuring.

10 **Continuously analyze aesthetic results.** Systematically compare standard before and after photos and solicit standardize patient comments. At the University of Pittsburgh, I have assisted in the development of a standardized deformity and outcome grading scale.

Chapter 5

Lower Body Reshaping

This chapter explores the lower portion of Total Body Lift surgery. The next several chapters detail the remaining components of body lift surgery. This compendium, available nowhere else, culminates in summary Chapter Ten. I offer this discourse because today's prospective patient has an insatiable appetite for information about plastic surgery. While Total Body Lift surgery can be performed in a single stage, most patients' usually complete body contouring in several stages, beginning with the lower body. The lower body extends from the umbilicus (navel) to below the knees.

Lower Body Weight Loss Deformity

"I can remember going to church on Easter praying, 'Dear Jesus, please don't give me legs like Aunt Linda.' She had these huge legs." – Laura

Massive weight loss leaves a spectrum of deformity. Body deflation relates to genetic specific fat depositions, skin elasticity, skin attachments to underlying muscles, muscular development, and skeletal form. The greater the change in body mass index (BMI) the more loose the skin deformity.

Lower body disorder is wrinkled and sagging skin of the back, abdomen, mons pubis, buttocks, and thighs. Skin rolls are partially emptied localized deposits of fat defined by horizontal adherence of dermis to deep fascia. Wrinkled skin is completely emptied of fat. Skin roll of an entire region or structure is considered ptosis. Swellings along the outer thighs are called saddlebags. As the skin loosens, the saddlebags become droopy. When the entire thighs were gigantic, then the loose and heavy remnant looked like pantaloons. The large lower abdominal skin and fat roll, overlapping the pubic and groin regions, is called a pannus. For the severely obese, the weighted pannus hangs to the knees and causes recurring infections. There may be a stack of rolls along the back and upper abdomen suggestive of the Michelin® tire man icon.

The skin neither looks nor feels right. We expect our skin to be adherent to our body, not floppy. The consistency is doughy. Many women shun touching their own skin or to be touched. The wobbly buttocks complicates sitting. Sitting is unstable, as if teetering on a Jell-O® mold. The excess skin bizarrely surrounds the thighs and buttocks like a life preserver.

Oversized people look normal, deflated people do not. The changed contour masculinizes women and feminizes men. The men are distressed by their hanging breasts. Their sagging thigh skin puckers, similar to the cellulite associated with women. Obese women resent the loss of their curvaceous femininity. Hips and thighs become square and the buttocks flat. Further fat loss leaves accordion like folds of skin hanging from boney prominences. Women despise their bizarrely drooping mons pubis, which obscures external genitalia. Coupled with unseemly rolls of inner thigh skin, these deformities may inhibit intimacy.

Overlapping skin traps moisture with increased microbe counts and mal odor, especially in the pubic region. Multiple daily cleansings are only a partial deterrent. Irritation lapses in to fungal growth and skin fold rashes. Proliferating skin bacterial flora can lead to cellulitis and abscesses. Flapping tissues thwart athletic activity. Hanging breasts and abdominal apron cause poor posture and painful back strain. Rolls of skin force a limited wardrobe of ill fitting clothes. Naked appearance becomes more objectionable than when obese. To illustrate my patient's perspective, let me introduce you to Sandra.

Sandra, a 37 year old mother of three toddlers, told me she despised her legs. She had lied about her weight for years. She was

5' 5" tall, yet she told people she was 5' 7" so that her weight seemed more in line with her height. As her BMI rose dangerously high, she was accepted for bariatric surgery. Her laparoscopic operation was a success. Over a year she effortlessly lost 110 pounds. Her dress size went from a size 22 to an 8. She had not felt so healthy during her entire adult life. She had gastric bypass surgery to be accepting of her body, yet afterwards she felt worse. She hid her belly, hips, and thighs under flowing pants. She was repulsed by her body odor, despite twice daily showers. Immediately before she went into the operating room, she said to me, "I don't care what the risks make me as tight as possible." During her lower body lift, abdominoplasty, and inner thigh lift, I pulled her skin as if fashioning a skin adherent leotard. She healed without problems, resulting in proportioned hips, flat abdomen, and most importantly firm inner thighs and shapely contoured outer thighs. Now Sandra parades into the office in shorts and skirts.

Lower body lifting is the most common surgical rehabilitation.

As they learn of the success of body contouring surgery, post-bariatric patients become increasingly intolerant of their bodies. Currently, about 20 percent of successful weight loss patients in Pittsburgh elect body contouring surgery. Lower body lifting is the most common surgical rehabilitation. Once all indicated surgical procedures are identified, a coordinated surgical plan is designed.

Circumferential abdominoplasty and lower body lift remove excess tissue and create feminine contours, leaving acceptable scars. **(See photo gallery, pages 1 and 2, for diagrams of incisions and scars)** I remove the skin between the umbilicus and pubis, including the hanging pannus. After exposing the upper central abdomen, I suture repair anterior abdominal fascial weakness and hernias. After lipoplasty of skin between the ribs and umbilicus, I pull it down over the lower abdominal wall to close the gap created by the panniculectomy. I continue the abdominoplasty around the lower back and buttocks into the lower body lift through a wide belt like excision between the waist and buttocks. Experience and good judgment is needed to access the appropriate amount of skin and not hazard excessive tension at closure. In most cases, to efface fully the saddlebag deformity, I need to undermine the thigh skin extensively and deeply. The undermining is by lipoplasty or long specialized instruments. Without undermining, the deep side of the skin is tethered to the muscular fascia, inhibiting upward lift.

While the upper inner thighs are slightly improved by the lower body lift, I prefer to add an inner thigh lift at the same time. At a minimum, a horizontal crescent of inner thigh is removed. By artfully extending the inner thigh excision along side of the mons pubis, complete correction of the ptotic mons is accomplished. Drooping of the mons pubis is corrected through these lateral skin excisions, extensive supra pubic excision, and lipoplasty. I can create a more attractive and tapered convex mound. The upper inner thighplasty does not correct skin redundancy below the mid thigh level. A vertical inner thighplasty is needed to address that region. A tapering band of excess inner thigh skin is removed from the pubis to the inner knee on each side.

The goal is to look good standing. Upright there is no skin distortion due to contact with a bed or chair. Hence, most surgeons map out pre-operatively with the patient standing. I agree that when the patient is standing, I can best determine if intended incisions lines are symmetrical and horizontal. Later while the patient is lying on the operating room table, the effects of gravity are changed and her own weight distorts nearby skin. Some surgeons plan excisions through a stenciled pattern. I prefer estimating excess skin by pushing, gathering, and pinching. The upper and lower incisions lie above and below the pinched together tissues. A helpful byproduct of comprehensive planning pre-operatively is the patient's full understanding of the operative plan. **NOTE: Refer to the patients in the photo gallery that have pre-operative markings.**

One of my innovations is novel incision planning. Contrary to mainstream thinking, I mostly mark the patient lying with her excess tissue pulled or suspended. The original reason was that these extremes of excess skin make standing pre-operative marking awkward and unreliable. Someone has to retract the hanging skin away just for me to see the region of interest. Ten pounds or more of pannus, thighs, and sagging buttocks are ungainly, making the magnitude of skin excision and final scar position uncertain. Comfortable with its accuracy, I have applied this marking technique to all body contouring situations.

Since the quality of incision healing is unpredictable, it is important to finish with the sutured closure under panties. Scar position relates to location, amount of excision, and the closure tension. As the patient lies on her back, she pulls up her abdominal skin with two hands, until the mons pubis is at the proper contour and tension. A 14 centimeter (six inch) horizontal line marks the upper border of the mons pubis centered eight centimeters (three inches) above the meeting of the Laba Majora. With the patient turned nearly on her side and opposite thigh slightly flex, the mons line is continued to the anterior superior iliac spine of the pelvis (forward boney prominence of the pelvis). After turning the patient completely on her side, an assistant supports the skyward leg. After I massage the loose thigh skin toward the bed, I can continue the line around the thigh on the way to the inter gluteal cleft.

This drawn circumferential line is the lower abdominal, hip hugging, and upper buttock incision. **(See photo gallery diagrams, pages 1, 2)** With this positioning we have taken advantage of gravity and not struggled against it. Because of the controlled tissue pulling and expectation of post-operative skin tensions from the thigh below and mid torso above, the final scar will reliably come to lie level along the bikini line. The photo gallery diagrams 1 and 2 have arrows that reflect the tension vectors (magnitude and direction of forces).

The upper circumferential abdominoplasty anticipated incision is drawn next. With her thigh rotated outward I place my hand along the hip portion of the lower incision and strongly slide upward toward the axilla (armpit). Excess skin is likewise dragged over my hand. A mark is made over my submerged fingertips. Tapering lines are drawn from this point to the umbilicus (navel) and the lower spine over the buttocks. This upper incision line demarcates the upper extent of skin removal. The circumferential band of skin removal looks like a broad belt as worn by a championship boxer.

The inner thigh skin excision lines are also drawn lying down. **(See photo gallery, page 8, of thigh drawing diagrams)** The skyward leg is abducted (thigh away from center) to mark the junction between the labia and thigh. Then after abducting the thigh (skyward leg centered) the mid thigh excess skin is massaged below the labia. I make a mid inner thigh lower mark. I draw a continuous line from the groin to that mark and then to the posterior lower buttock thigh crease. I remove all the skin between these two lines in the form of a crescent. When we wish to treat a thigh-long severe deformity I plan a vertical excision inner thigh extension to the knee. **(See photo gallery, page 9, of thigh drawing diagrams)** As the vertical inner thighplasty leaves a visible scar down the thigh, the incisions are placed through tissue gathering techniques so that the final scar lies towards the back of the inner thigh. After all these incision lines are made in multiple positions in the bed, the lines are adjusted with the patient standing. **(See photo gallery, pages 1, 2)**

Positioning

Correcting a circumferential deformity requires at least one complete turn of the patient. For decades I was comfortable performing body lifts by starting in the prone position and then turning supine. In the 1990s, luminary surgeon Ted Lockwood from Kansas City convinced me and many others to change that method to side to side lateral positioning, ending supine. He is renowned for redesigning the inner thighplasty and improving the lower body lift. He is a superb teacher, presenting outstanding results. Applying his three positions to the oversized massive weight loss patient was awkward, restrictive, and inefficient. Hence, I returned to the simpler prone and supine positioning. To optimize the prone position I had to again innovate. This time it was full thigh abduction onto a side table.

This technical innovation relates to surgical principles 2 and 8 at the end of the last chapter. The loose skin deformity is diffuse. The removal of hanging skin leaves still abnormally lax skin. The remaining inelastic skin will stretch over a short period of time leading to recurrent but smaller saddlebags. Removal of as much skin as possible followed by a high-tension closure of the skin flaps minimizes this problem. A tight closure occurs when the approximated skin is fully stretched, like the parchment over the banjo's circular body. Over some weeks the skin will give some and the tension will be natural. The skin will be tightest when standing and the legs are together. When the legs are spread apart the incision closure is not so tight. Since closure should not be performed with excessive tension, I take advantage of flexion across the lateral thigh by moving the leg outward (abduction) when closing along the hips.

By favorably positioning the leg outward in the prone position, the hip saddlebag deformity can be corrected under less tension than when the legs are together. Early in my experience, the outward positioning of the legs was limited to the width of the operating room table. An operating table is fairly narrow at two and a half feet so that favorable positioning was restricted. I was perplexed that I could not move the leg out wider. The advantage of the lateral or sideways position was that the upper leg could be raised up on cushions to narrow the wound gap for closure. The disadvantages of that positioning were the limited access and unstable footing on top of cushions. I imagined that if the leg were pulled out in space that the closure would be expedited.

I conceived that a small, padded utility table could be moved alongside the main OR table, and with the help of the circulating nurse, we could pull out the leg and safely place it there. This is similar to the common maneuver of placing the arm on an arm board extension for hand surgery. Over my 25 years of practicing plastic surgery, I have never moved the leg off the table. When the leg is fully abducted on to this table more skin can be removed than previously possible. This position now allows tension free suturing of the undersurface of the lateral thigh skin to deep muscle to close the dissected space. After large towel clips, which look like miniature ice tongs, squeeze the skin flaps together, the two layer skin suturing is done under no tension. Lately I have been abducting the leg on to a well padded articu-lating arm board, which is a little less cumbersome than moving in the side table. One of the advantages of the prone position is that when the closure is completed, the first leg is returned to the straight position on the operating table. This extraordinarily tight skin along the lateral thigh corrects the saddlebag deformity, raises the buttock, and smoothes out the upper anterior (front) thigh.

I could see that my results were better, but I wanted to prove that scientifically. My colleagues at the University of Pittsburgh joined me to meticulously and independently study my clinical outcomes. We organized sets of standardized before and after photographs, using the new leg positioning, and compared them to a similar set without the innovation. We devised and implemented a grading scale. Mathematical statistics validated significant improvement in the correction of the saddlebag deformity as well as contours of the mons pubis. (Hurwitz, D.J., Rubin J. P., Risen M., Sejjadian A., Serieka, S.., Correcting the Saddlebag deformity in the Massive Weight Loss Patient, *Plastic and Recon. Surgery* 114:5;1313-1325, October, 2004) That was a series of about 30 patients. I am still making further improvements to the technique, but the results stand.

At the start of the operation, my patient is induced under general anesthesia on the pre-operative cart. After the breathing (endotrachial) tube is placed she is turned prone onto the operating room table, covered with sterile sheets. Her face is cradled in a special foam rubber cut out pillow. The lower body lift is started through the lower incision, first the left side then the right. Because the prone position allows me to see the entire back and buttocks, I am better able to achieve a level transverse scar. The prone position facilitates team surgery, which also shortens operative time without sacrificing quality.

Optimum surgeon position facilitates any procedure, but it is particularly important in body contouring. This seemingly mundane facet of complex surgery is often ignored even by seasoned practitioners. The position of the surgeon is to some extent a personal matter, depending on whether he or she is right or left handed, visual focal length, agility, and size. Total Body Lift surgery is physically demanding with long hours standing and forceful retraction of heavy tissues. Thought should be given to physical comfort and good visibility. I remind my trainees that surgery has similarities to sexual intercourse; in both, position counts a lot and better performed when effectively using both hands. When several operators can close wounds created by the surgeon, then positioning, timing, and movement around the table can be optimally choreographed.

As the operation begins with elevation of the loose lower body, I stand at the right side of the prone torso. My working right hand can advance easily into the tissues as my helping left hand retracts nearby tissues. Skilled assistants are counter retracting for proper exposure. As one surgeon suture closes the left back and flank, I and another assistant remove excess tissue from the right side. After that area is prepared for closure by my assistants, I move across the table to the patient's left knee to remove excess skin from under the buttock folds. If a long broad excision vertical thigh lift is planned then the posterior incision is made. If a contemporaneous upper body lift is to be done, then I move up to the left side and remove a mid back swath of skin. Finally, I return to the right side back and create an identical back wound. Both back wounds are then closed.

At the completion of the prone portion of the procedure, the back, hips, and upper thighs have been closed in two layers of strong suture. The side wounds are left open to be closed later when the patient is in the supine position. The anesthetized patient is prepared for turning over by wrapping a sterile surgeon's gown around her like a cocoon. While wrapped in a gown, she is gently picked up and rolled over onto a second table. The gown is opened up with the patient face up and imme-diately ready for reprep with antiseptic, lying on a water imper-meable sterile field. My turn procedure increases ease, safety and sterility for an otherwise awkward maneuver.

I stand along side her right hip to finish the lower abdomino-plasty incision. After removing the excess skin, I sutured tight the central muscular fascia. I confirm the amount of skin to be removed between the umbilicus and pubis and then remove it. After I align the remaining flaps for closure and create a central triangular opening for the umbilicoplasty, I take an assistant down to the thighs. Now lower down on the right side of the table, I remove skin for the inner thighplasty and mons pubicplasty. Meanwhile assistants are closing the lower abdomen under my supervision. After I secure the raised skin to the deep tissues of the pubic region, an assistant closes the skin, allowing me to move up to the right side of her chest to complete the upper body lift and breast reshaping. A complete description of this part of the operation was published in *Seminars in Plastic Surgery*, Number 3, August 2004; Breast Reshaping after Massive Weight Loss, pages 179 to 187.

Suzanne's Story

After dieting off 55 pounds and another surgeon performed lipoplasty, 38 year old Suzanne complained about loose lower body skin. She lamented that "I had to tuck my rolls of flab back into my clothes when I got dressed. When I jogged, my excess skin flapped all over." Since she would not return to sports and exercising at the gym, she was regaining her weight. After an abdominoplasty and lower body lift, Suzanne wears shorts and skirts with confidence. She attends lunch hour aerobics class and works out with a trainer four times a week. She is more physically active and her body is more toned than when she was in her twenties.

Summery of Lower Body Lift Operation Only

The operation begins with the infusion of large volumes of dilute epinephrine to minimize bleeding. I remove excess fat by

Photo Gallery

The diagrams in this gallery are borrowed from my scientific presentations. They assist in understanding the planning and performance of Total Body Lift surgery. The before and after photographs of recent body contouring operations were graciously allowed by my patients. I thank them for their cooperation. I selected these cases to demonstrate the broad range of deformities and their treatment. All patients are pleased with their remarkable, but at times incomplete improvement. None required emergency reoperation or hospitalization. Most had minor healing problems that improved with dressing care. Understandably I have avoided name identification, except that patients in the gallery quoted in the book are so cited. For a modicum of modesty the nipples and labia are covered.

Photo Gallery page 1 TOTAL BODY LIFT frontal diagrams. Three diagrams of planning, treatment and scars of Total Body Lift Surgery in the front view. (Left) The lines of the upper body lift include reshaping a saging breast and removal of mid torso roll. The abdominoplasty removes the abdominal apron. The loose medial thigh is to be corrected by drawn vertical thighplasty. (Middle) The broad belt excision of skin is indicated in red. The deepithelization of the breast is indicated in yellow. The vector closure tensions are indicated by the arrows. As the vectors indicate the greatest tension of closure is lateral (to the sides) (Left) The final scar position is seen in faint red along the bikini and bra lines and just back of the mid inner line of the thighs.

Photo Gallery page 2 TOTAL BODY LIFT back diagrams. Three diagrams of planning, treatment and scars of Total Body Lift surgery in the back view. (Left) A broad band removes mid torso roll. The abdominoplasty removes the abdominal apron. The loose medial thigh is to be corrected by drawn vertical thighplasty. (Middle) The broad belt excision of skin is indicated in red. The deepithelization of the back flaps for the breasts is indicated in yellow. The vector closure tensions are indicated by the arrows. As the vectors indicate the greatest tension of closure is lateral (to the sides) (Left) The final scar position is seen in faint red along the bikini and bra lines.

Photo Gallery page 3 These are before (personal snap shot) and after clothed photos of a 34 year old who had Laparoscopic Roux en-Y bypass followed three years later by my Total Body Lift with L brachioplasties. Her initial weight was 335 pounds and she now weighs 145 (BMI 50 to 28). She owns a beauty shop. She married her sweetheart Greg several months after her last operation. Medical reporter Marilyn Brooks of Pittsburgh's WTAE TV (an ABC affiliate) told her story on the evening news during February 2004. See a portion on www.hurwitz-center.com. One year after her Lift I also augmented her breasts and performed vertical medial thighplasties.

Photo Gallery pages 4 & 5 These are pre- and one year post-operative views of the woman, seen on the last page. Her first operation was an abdominoplasty, lower body lift, inner thighplasty with L brachioplasties. I removed 18 pounds during her body lift. Eight months later I performed breast augmentation with saline filled implants and vertical thighplasties. Her heavy large arms, multiple rolls of mid torso skin, and sagging lower body and thighs were corrected. She was featured in my article on Single Stage Total Body Lift Surgery in the *Annals of Plastic Surgery*, also found on www.hurwitzcenter.com.

Photo Gallery page 6 At 58 years and weighing 318 pounds, she had Laparoscopic Roux en-Y bypass. Fourteen months and 188 pounds later, she had multistaged Total Body Lift (abdominoplasty, lower body lift, vertical thighplasty, and upper body lift with breast reshaping using local flaps) and L brachioplasties. She suffered from extreme loose skin of her thighs. I removed further skin on the inner and outer thigh on two more occasions.

Photo Gallery page 7 56 year old woman 5' 6", weighing 153 pounds desired smaller breasts and an overall improved shape in her body. I reduced her 38 DD cup sized breasts to 36 C. She had a Brazilian abdominoplasty, with bands of skin remove above her pubis and groins, and below her breasts. Her back and hips were sculptured with Vaser® LipoSelection℠ to achieve a well proportioned curvaceous figure. The results are seen six months later as the scars are beginning to fade.

Photo Gallery page 8 This is a three part diagram of marking an upper inner thighplasty. (top) In this view of her bottom, the patient raises her left leg outward. As my assistant pushes the loose thigh skin towards the knee, I draw the upper incision line between her labia majora and thigh. (Middle) The point of maximal skin resection along the middle of the inner thigh is determined with the thigh moved inward. I push all loose skin downward. At the level of the labia majora, I mark the smoothed thigh skin lower limit of resection. (bottom) As the thigh is again held out I extend a crescent shaped inferior incision line from this inferior resection mark to the pubic region in the front and the buttock thigh junction line in the back.

Photo Gallery page 9 This sequence of diagrams is the vertical excision band extension to the knee. (top) With the leg on the bed, and superior and medial drag on the anterior thigh skin, I draw the front excision line from the inner knee up the thigh to the apex of the previously drawn crescent excision line. (middle) I gather the width of maximal resection at the mid thigh and mark this point back of the front excision line. (bottom) From this mid thigh mark, I drew a widening back incision line from below knee to the ischial tuberosity (sitting bone). I adjust the entire excision backward, moving the closure back so it cannot be seen in the standing position. The final scar forms an L shape.

Photo Gallery page 10 (top) This diagram shows removal of the vertical excision band along the inner thigh. After checking the accuracy of the width in the frog leg position, I start near the near the knee to cut out the excess skin and fat of the entire inner thigh down to thigh muscles. (middle) The leg is moved in from the frog leg position to accurately determine the extent of upper crescent excision. After the excess skin is excised, large braided sutures anchors the thigh skin flap to the pubic bone. The skin is closed in two more layers of sutures. (bottom) This is a drawing of the completed closure which resembles an L than curves from the thigh to the ischial tuberosity (sitting bone) and then ascends between the thigh and labia to the groin.

Photo Gallery page 11 This sequence of photos is the before and one year after lower body lift and vertical thighplasties in a 46 year old 5' 5" tall, 170 pound woman who had lost 227 pounds following gastric bypass. She had the worst lower body and thigh skin excess that I have treated. Only a small amount of residual excess skin around the knees distracts from an amazing result. The last before picture shows the immediate preoperative markings. Notice how wide the skin removal is along her lower torso and thighs. She was featured in my article on the saddlebag deformity in the October 2004 issue of the *Journal of Plastic and Reconstructive Surgery*.

Photo Gallery page 12 This sequence of photos is the before and one year after single stage Total Body Lift surgery. After losing 130 pounds through dieting and exercise, this 23 year old web designer desired breast, abdominal, hip, and thigh body contouring. Her greatest concern was her "old lady breasts." I raised and slightly reduced her breasts, an abdominoplasty, lower body lift and upper inner thighplasty, which was taped by Discovery Health Channel November 2003. Her story called "Deluxe contour" played on *Plastic Surgery Before and After* program throughout 2004 and into 2005. Portions can be viewed on www.hurwitzcenter.com. She was featured on the January 3, 2005 cover story on massive weight loss by dieting in *People Magazine*, which earned her an appearance on NBC's Jane Pauley show. She says, "I owe my self confidence to this surgery."

Photo Gallery page 13 This sequence of photos is the before and two years after two stage Total Body Lift surgery, followed by limited scar revisions. This 137 pound, 5' 4" 27 year old lost 180 pounds after gastric bypass surgery. She married six months after her last operation and is three months pregnant in her after photos. Her first operation was an abdominoplasty, lower body lift, vertical thighplasty, and breast lift with saline implant augmentation. Her second operation was an upper body lift with revision of her breast reshaping and bilateral brachioplasties.

Photo Gallery page 14 This sequence of photos is the before and 6 months after one stage Total Body Lift (abdominoplasty, inner thigh lift, lower body lift, upper body lift, breast reshaping with local flaps). She is 5' 8" and went from 370 pounds to 225 pounds after gastric bypass surgery. She was at least 20 pounds more than desirable; I nevertheless did a single stage Total Body Lift with removal of 18 pounds of skin and fat. She has gained some of that back, but remains pleased with her improved feminine contours. Her story was featured on ABC national television Deborah Norvell's "Inside Edition" during April 2004. See portions on www.hurwitzcenter.com. She is an elementary school teacher who is proud that her little students like her transformation.

Photo Gallery pages 15 & 16 This sequence of photos is the before and one year after one stage Total Body Lift (abdominoplasty, inner thigh lift, lower body lift, upper body lift, breast reshaping with local flaps) and brachioplasties in a 41 year old. She is a married accountant, who lost 150 pounds after minimally invasive gastric bypass surgery. She despised her bat wing like arms. Her operation took eight hours. She received no blood transfusions and was discharged from the hospital two days later. Her early return to work in two weeks is unusually fast. Her story and surgery was presented by medical reporter Marilyn Brooks on WTAE news (a Pittsburgh, ABC affiliate) in May 2004 and a portion can be seen on www.hurwitzcenter.com.

Photo Gallery page 17 An extended keyhole shaped pattern is drawn which includes excess upper abdominal skin and fat below the breast as well as the back roll to the side. The side flap ends near the tip of the scapula (shoulder blade). (Top right). All flap extensions are deepithelialized (skinned) and elevated from the muscles (Bottom left). The upper abdominal flap is folded on itself to augment the inferior breast. The lateral extension spirals around the breast to fit into a tunnel between the breast and muscle. (Bottom right) The reshaped and augmented breast with deepthelialized flaps in place.

Photo Gallery page 18 This sequence of photos is the before and two years after two stage Total Body Lift surgery and brachioplasties in a 5' 6", 220 pound 49 year old. At 510 pounds she was home bound. She lost 280 pounds after open gastric bypass surgery but is immobilized by her excess skin. She hated both her hanging abdomen and thighs. She preferred not to have breast implants. In the first stage she had abdominoplasty, lower body lift, upper inner thighplasty. In the second stage four months later she had an upper body lift with breast reshaping using local flap augmentation and vertical thighplasties. She is accepted to veterinary school.

Photo Gallery page 19 This sequence of photos is the before and two years after two stage Total Body Lift surgery and brachioplasties in a 5' 6", 190 pound 56 year old. She lost 120 pounds after open gastric bypass, which also left her with a large mid abdominal incisional hernia. In stage one I repaired the hernia during an abdominoplasty, lower body lift and upper inner thigh lift. Six months later she had an upper body lift with breast reductions and bilateral brachioplasties. Some months later she some scar revisions and a facelift. She gained about 20 pounds since her last surgery, but is pleased with her results. She was featured in my article on Single Stage Total Body Lift in the *Annals of Plastic Surgery*, May 2004, available on www.hurwitzcenter.com.

Photo Gallery page 20 This sequence of photos is the before and 8 months after one stage Total Body Lift with correction of bilateral gynecomastia with extensive use of ultrasonic assisted lipoplasty. He is 6' 1" 180 pounds, having lost over 100 pounds from gastric bypass surgery. He reframed for beach or intimacy until I corrected his skin excess and sagging breasts.

Photo Gallery page 21 This sequence of photos is the before and 6 months after one stage Total Body Lift with correction of bilateral gynecomastia using my boomerang excision technique. He is 5' 11" 190 pounds, having lost over 100 pounds from open gastric bypass surgery. While troubled by his hanging abdominal apron, it was his sagging breasts that troubled him the most. He never exposed his chest in public. Following abdominoplasty, lower body lift, upper inner thigh-plasty, I corrected his gynecomastia with removal of excess tissue and upward positioning of his nipples. He now goes shirtless on the beach.

Photo Gallery page 22 This sequence of photos is the before and one year after one stage Total Body Lift (abdominoplasty, inner thigh lift, lower body lift, upper body lift, breast reshaping with local flaps) in a 49 year old married woman. She is 5' 6" and weighs160 pounds, having lost 150 after minimally invasive gastric bypass surgery. She hated her loose thighs and sagging breasts and loved the improvement. She then focused on her severely sagging arms face and neck. Five months later, her second set of operations were facelift, endoscopic assisted brow lift, and bilateral L brachioplasty.

Photo Gallery page 23 These photos were taken of the 49 year old woman who had Total Body Lift surgery shown on the prior page. She is just before her bypass surgery and three months after her facelift, brow lift, and brachioplasties more confident than ever, but a little con-cerned that old friends do not recognize her.

Photo Gallery page 24 This sequence of photos is the before and six weeks after one stage Total Body Lift (abdominoplasty, inner thigh lift, lower body lift, upper body lift, breast reshaping with local flaps) in a 44 year old 5' 5" married woman. She had minimally invasive gastric bypass three years before, loosing 120 pounds down to 140. She admits to low self esteem because of her hanging skin of the abdomen and thighs. She received two units of blood and was discharged three days after her body lift. She demonstrates excellent early healing and body contour soon after major surgery. There is still some swelling and these early scars are red and will soon fade.

Photo Gallery page 25 This sequence of photos is the before and one week after her MACS (Minimal Access Cranial Suspension) facelift and silicone chin implant. These procedures were performed in my office operating room with minimal sedation under three hours. These early after photos show how little swelling and bruising occurs after this less invasive facelift procedure. She returned to nursing ten days after her facelift, which was seven weeks after her Total Body Lift. Very please with the results, her self confidence has soared. Her story will be on "Plastic Surgery Before and After" on Discovery Health Cable in 2005.

Photo Gallery page 26 This sequence of photos is the before and one year after three stage Total Body Lift surgery and brachioplasties in a 5' 3", 170 pound 47 year old. She weighed over 400 pounds prior to her minimally invasive gastric bypass surgery. Her first stage Total Body Lift was an abdominoplasty, lower body lift and vertical inner thigh-plasty. Three months later, her second stage was an upper body lift with breast reshaping using mastopexy. Four months later she had bilateral L brachioplasties and minor revisions of past procedures. While still a full sized woman, she is thrilled with the loss of her hanging skin and the creation of voluptuous contours.

Photo Gallery pages 27 & 28 This sequence of photos is the before and one year after single stage Total Body Lift surgery and bra-chioplasties in a 5' 3", 158 pound 41 year old. She weighed 350 pounds before her minimally invasive gastric bypass. She is thrilled by the result, especially the improvement in her massive upper arms. She developed a left side abdominal laparoscopic incision hernia. Soon I will repair her hernia and remove some residual excess of her abdomen. She happily told her success story on the Jennifer Annkowiak morning show on Pittsburgh's KDKA- TV (a CBS affiliate) July 2004.

Photo Gallery page 29 This sequence of photos is the before and four months after single stage Total Body Lift surgery (abdominoplasty, lower body lift, limited vertical thighplasties, upper body lift with breast reshaping using local flaps) and brachioplasties in a 5' 5", 170 pound 48 year old married woman. She also had an uncomplicated course and returned to work in the food service industry within two months of her surgery.

Photo Gallery page 30 This sequence of photos is the before and one year after single stage Total Body Lift surgery (abdominoplasty, lower body lift, inner thighplasty and breast reshaping with silicone gel implants) in a 5' 5", 130 pound 32 year old. She weighed 350 pounds and lost her excess weight by dieting. Within a year she was married and recently delivered her first baby. She was on the cover of *People Magazine* May 2004.

Photo Gallery page 31 This sequence of photos is the before and two years after three stage Total Body Lift surgery and brachioplasties in a 5' 3", 200 pound 55 year old woman. She had lost 90 pounds through dieting and exercise. Her first stage was an upper body lift with breast reshaping and bilateral brachioplasties. Five months later, her second stage was an abdominoplasty, lower body lift and inner thighplasty. The result is seen in the middle photo. Six months later further liposuction and scar revision was done and the early result is in the last photo.

Photo Gallery page 32 This sequence of photos is the before and a years after single stage Total Body Lift surgery (abdominoplasty, lower body lift, inner thighplasties, ultrasonic assisted lipoplasty and short scar mastopexies) in a 5' 5", 135 pound 43 year old married woman with a 23 year old son. Despite vigorous exercise, she could never restore her abdominal shape. She was disheartened by her sagging breasts. She is thrilled with the results and work out daily to maintain her sensuous figure.

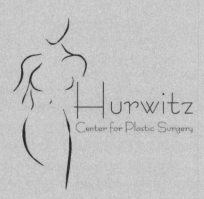

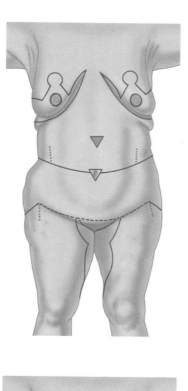

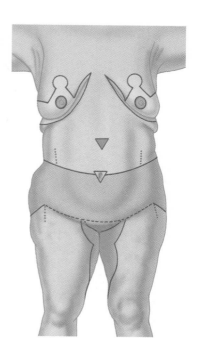

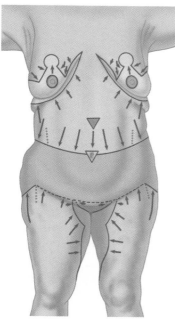

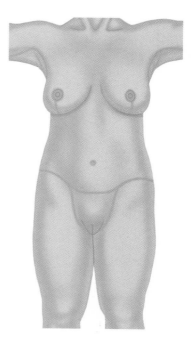

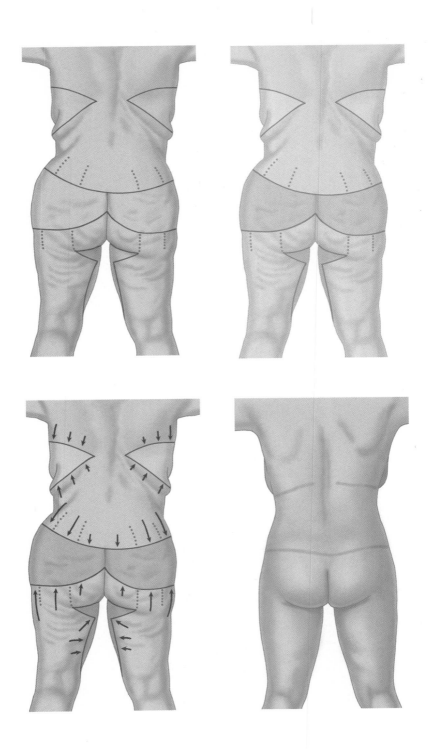

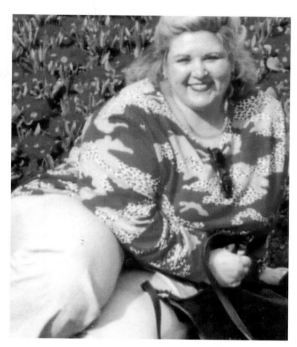

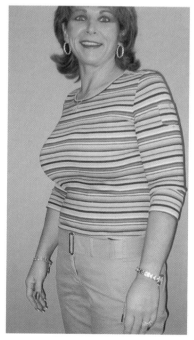

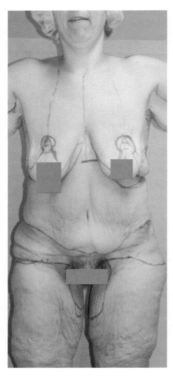

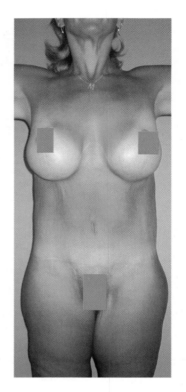

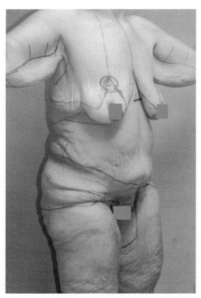

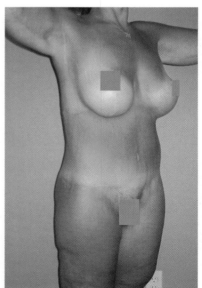

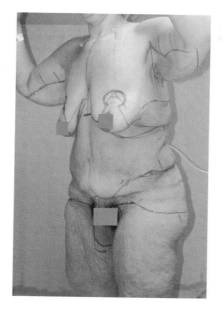

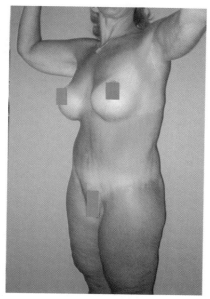

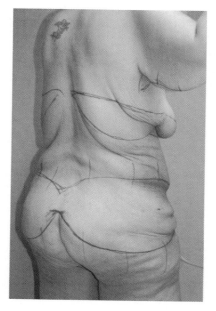

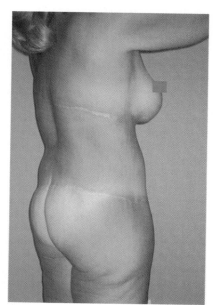

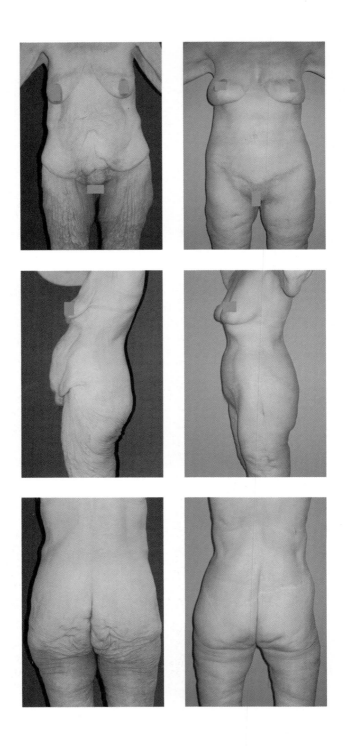

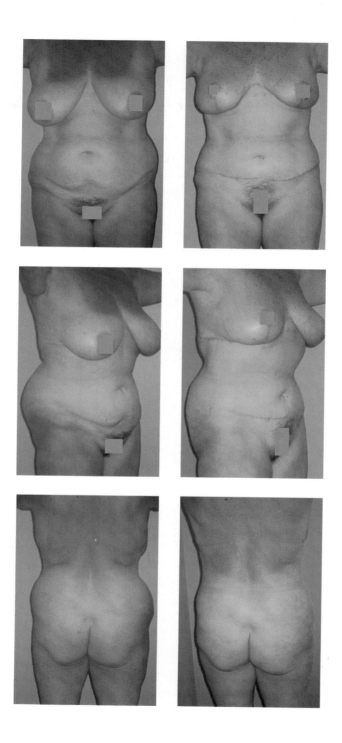

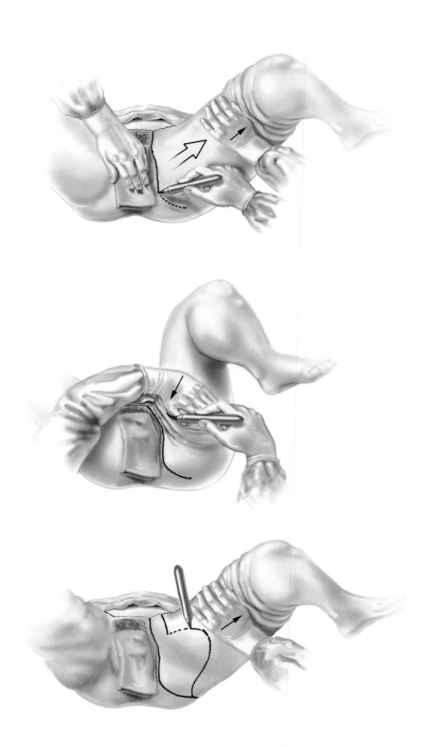

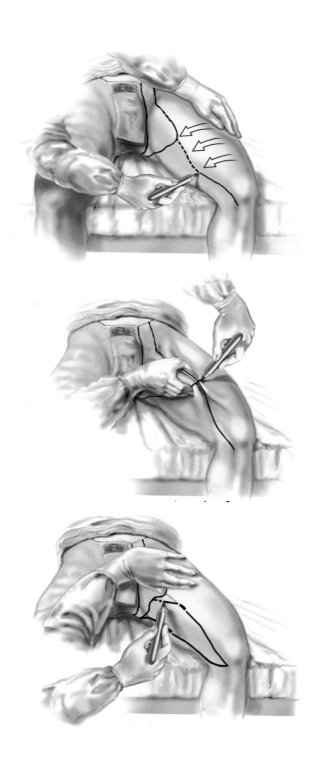

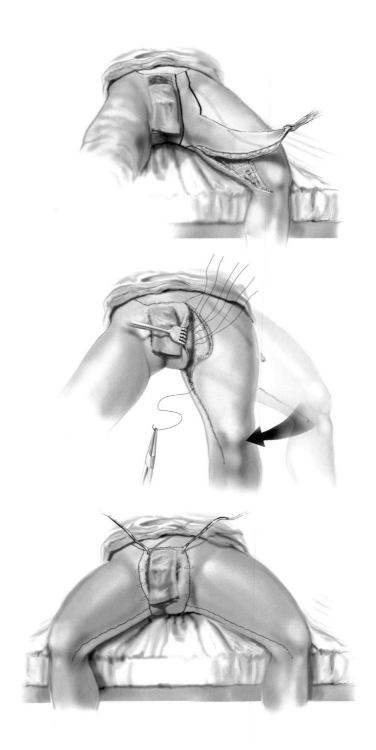

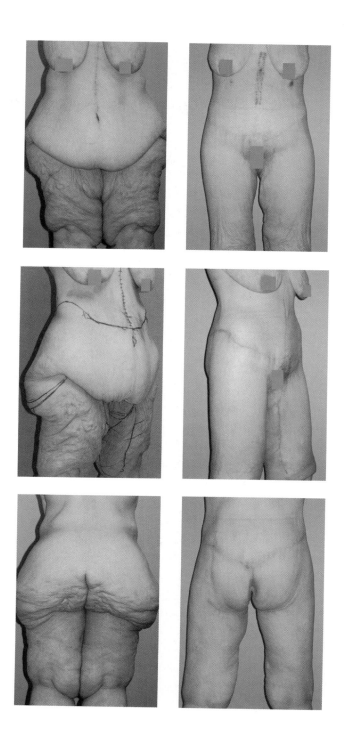

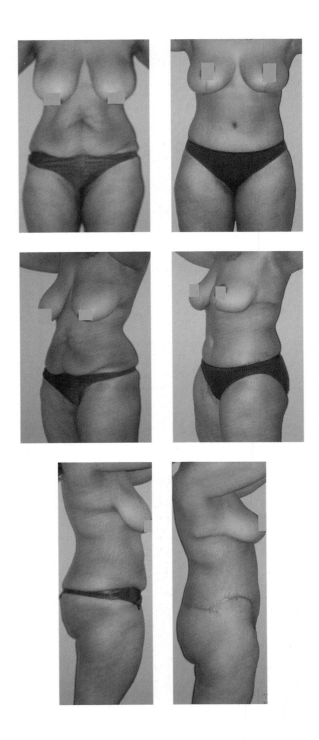

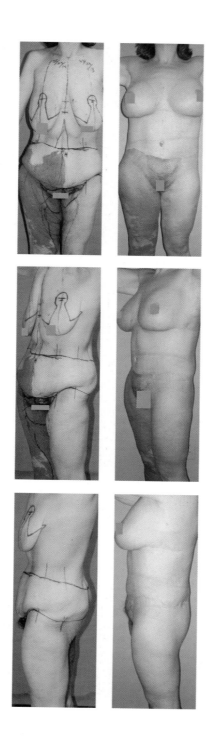

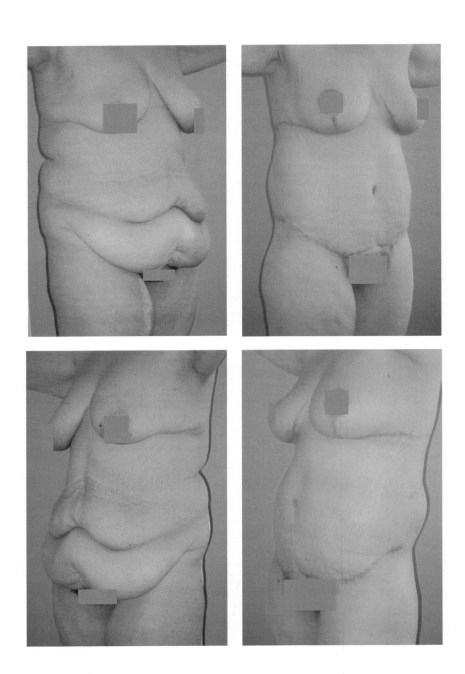

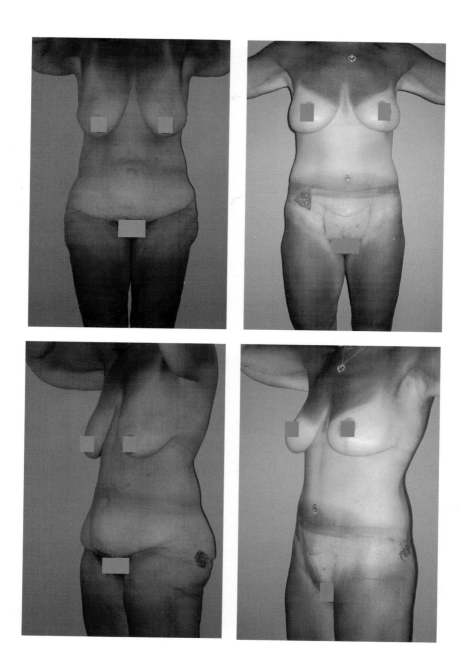

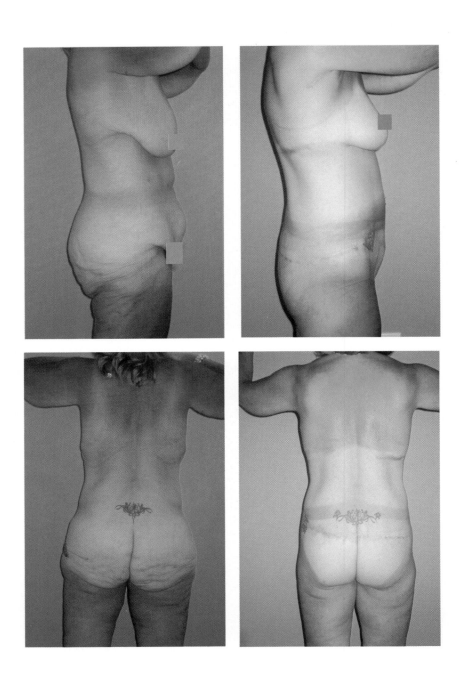

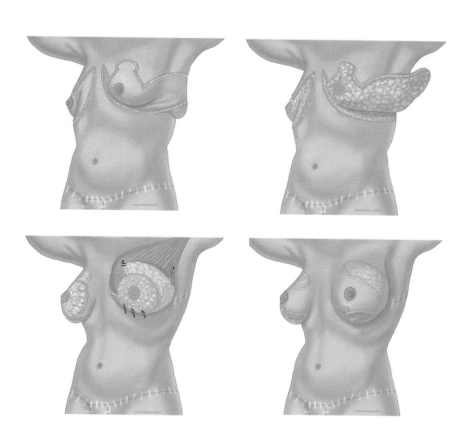

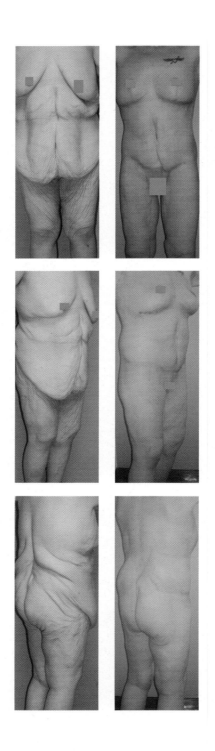

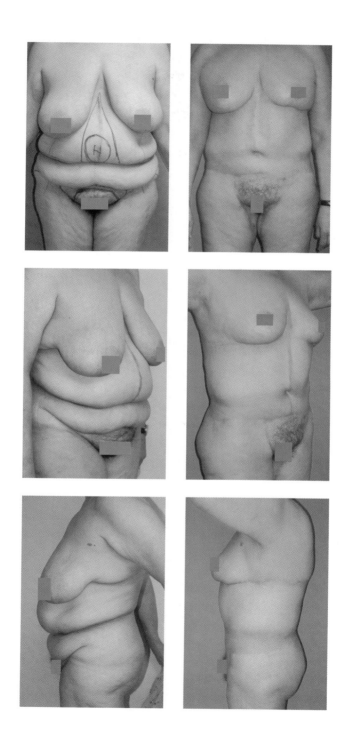

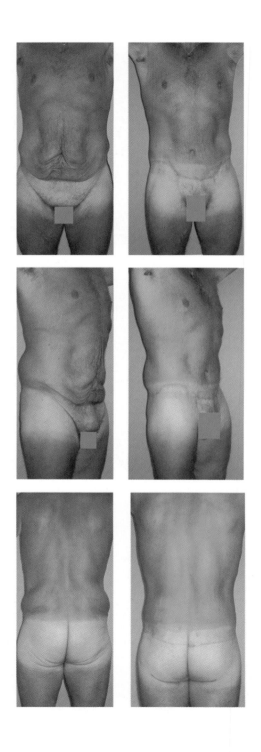

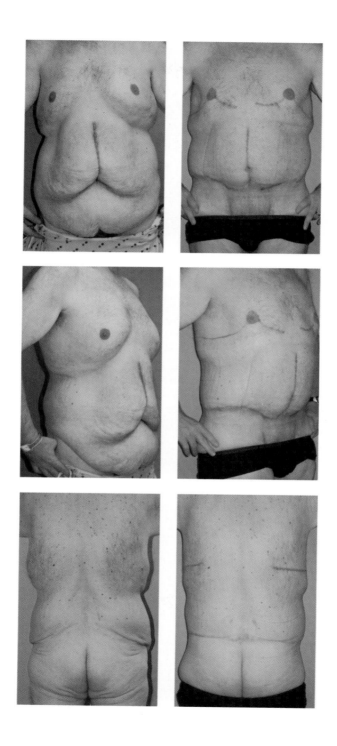

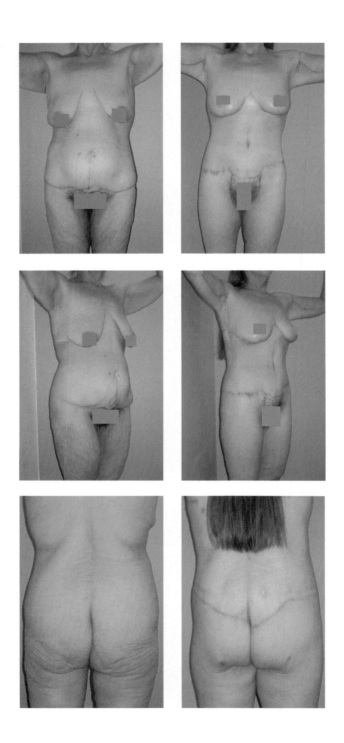

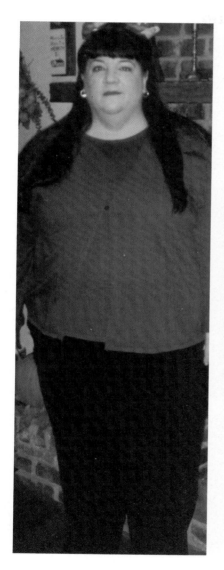
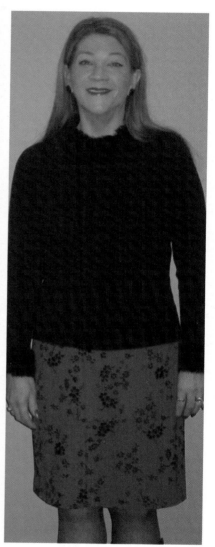

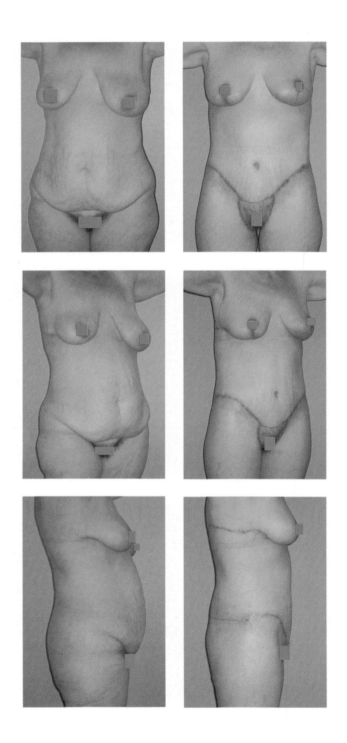

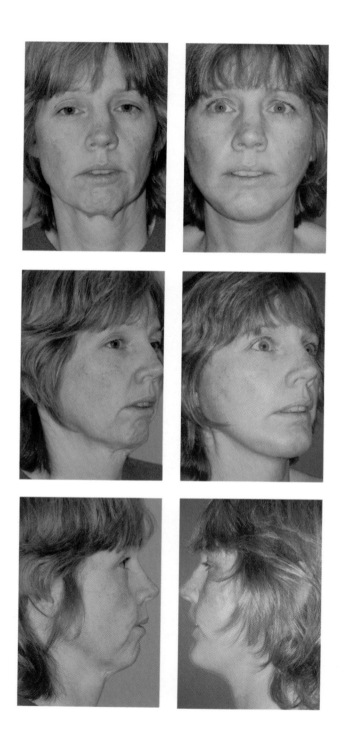

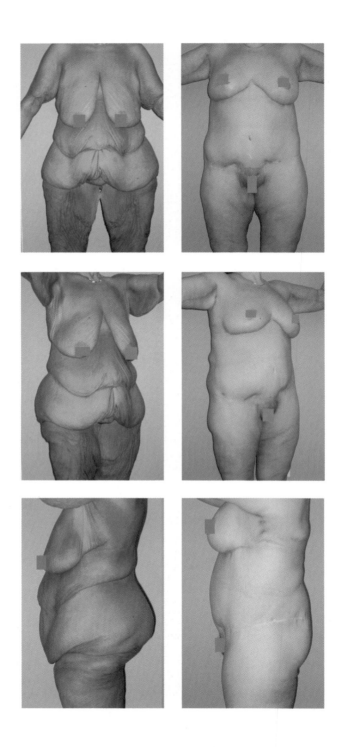

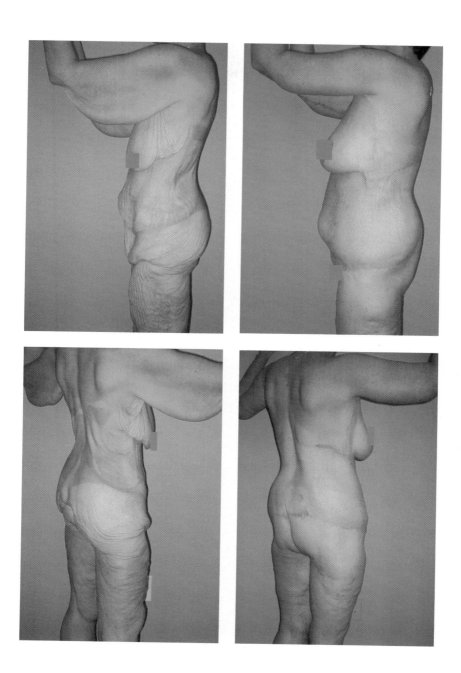

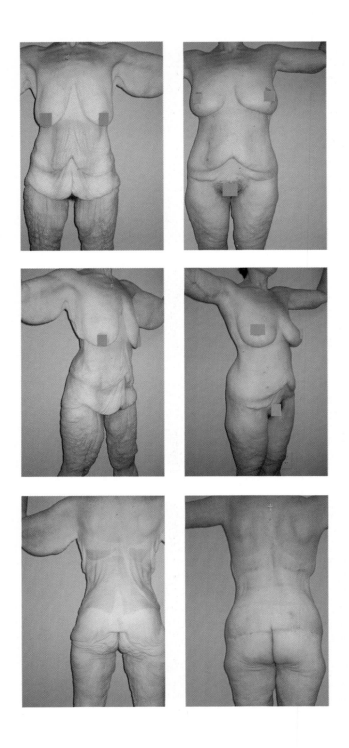

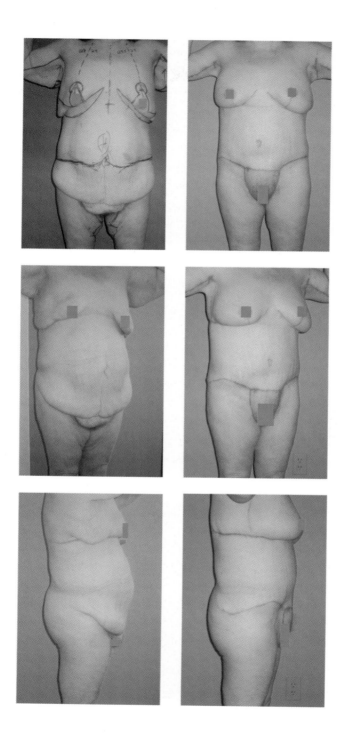

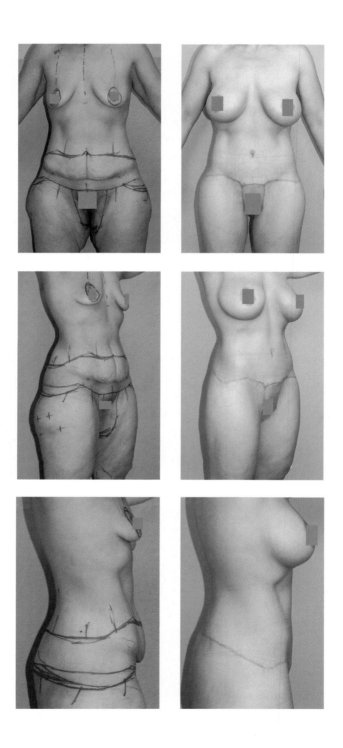

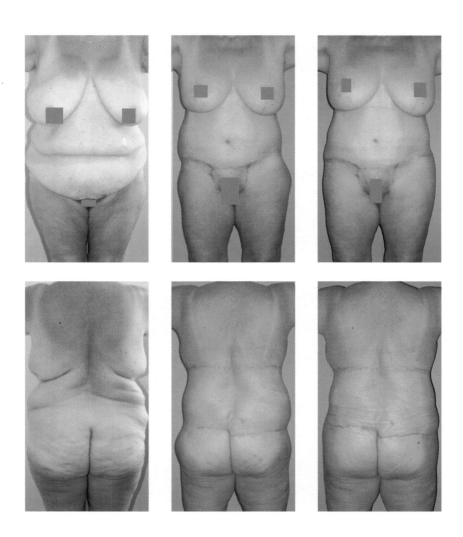

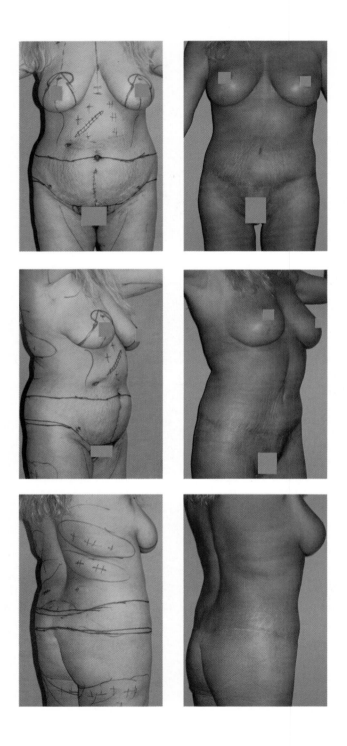

LipoSelection℠. I incise the lower back and hips along the lower transverse incision line through the skin and fat. I mobilize the buttock and thigh skin. I pull this skin upwards and the intended superior incision line along the waist is confirmed and cut. Then this belt like band of skin between these two incisions is removed, taking care to leave behind an appropriate amount of fat for better contour. I fully abduct the left leg to facilitate skin closure. While the left flank and lower back is being closed, a matching procedure is performed on her right side. Before I turn her over, I resect some of the inner thigh skin under her buttocks and close the small wounds.

After the turn, I continue the abdominoplasty across the groins and over the pubis. I raise abdominal skin flap over the muscular fascia to just above the upper transverse incision line. I remove the excess skin between the umbilicus (navel) and pubis, leaving a dime sized triangular island of umbilicus (navel). I then undermine midline skin between the lower chest and umbilicus to pull the upper flap down to the pubis. I plicate the midline fascia, which means that I fold it on itself with sutures. With moderate flexion of the trunk, I close the abdominoplasty and residual lower body lift. I deliver the umbilical skin triangle through a similar triangular opening, like a button through a new button hole. Finally, I remove excess inner thigh skin and I hitch up sagging inner thigh subcutaneous fascia to either side of the pubic bone for tension free closure of the thigh to labial skin.

Special Challenges

Since there is little margin for error between a tight, secure closure and a tight closure that splits, problems in healing can occur. Some minor separations have occurred. If caught early they respond to bedside suturing. Later, the wounds heal in with dressing care. Those scars are likely to need revision. Some primary healed scars become hypertrophic or raised, due to genetic tendency or excessive tension.

The most common problem is seroma. After the drainage tubes are removed the serum weeping may resume beyond the capability of the tissue to absorb, leaving puddles or collections of fluid. These early seromas respond well to repeated syringe aspirations. Sometimes, we insert a new suction drain for a week.

Pubic Monsplasty

The mons pubis is sensual, curvaceous fullness of haired skin above the pubic bone. Flanked on each side by the valleys of the hairless groins, the mons is derived from the lower abdomen and flows into the subtle convexity of the labia majora. The mons pubis is distorted by weight loss and surgical scars. The youthful mons is convex and vertical. The aged mons is flat and horizontal. Women hate mons pubis ptosis. They will not wear hip hugging pants, bathing suits, or be seen nude.

This droopiness is only partially treated with other techniques. I have had uniform success with a three-sided picture frame excision. The topside of the picture frame is a tight abdominoplasty, an essential first step to properly shape the mons. Many surgeons stop there with incomplete results. I have added the two sides of the picture frame excision to stretch out and support the sagging structure. These two- to three-inch wide groin skin excisions are continuous with the previously performed inner thighplasty. By keeping the side skin excision very thin, problematic prolonged swelling of the pubic area due to interruption of lymphatics is avoided. Lipoplasty flattens the oversized mound and sensation is maintained. The ideal result leaves a gentle convexity from the umbilicus to the junction of the labia majora. My patients have reported less inhibition and improved sex.

This same technique can be modified to revise an inadequate first monsplasty. In fact, after adapting a three sided picture frame approach for revisions, I realized what a powerful tool I had for the initial operation.

Challenges

If the closure between the mons and abdomen is too tight, the deep suture closure may spread leaving a depression. The most severe sagging may not be correctable and a second stage may be needed. This area is prone to hypertrophic scars.

Vertical Thighplasty

Exceptionally loose and even heavy tissues throughout the thighs are a common problem after massive weight loss. The traditional upper inner thighplasty that I just described cannot deal with this deformity. I find a vertical thighplasty indicated in many patients. Not only does it improve the aesthetics of the thigh, but the thighplasty eliminates excessive pulling on the bikini scar line of the lower body lift.

The vertical thighplasty builds on the upper inner thighplasty by including a wide band of skin along the entire length of the thigh. The optimum location is from the inner side of the knee to the back portion of the labia. The excision is a vertical strip up the thigh. (See diagrams in photo gallery, pages 9, 10) It leaves a long scar, which lies along the inner aspect, toward the backside. In that location the scar is not seen with the legs reasonably close together. (See photo gallery, page 11) Ultimately the scar is faint and acceptable. A complete description of the medial thighplasty is published in the *Aesthetic Surgery Journal*. (Hurwitz D.J. Medial Thighplasty for Operative Strategies, *Aesthetic Society Journal* accepted for March-April 2005 issue)

Challenges

Occasionally healing can be delayed near the labia or the knee. The problem near the labia is small areas of skin loss and separation of closures, which need to be cleaned and allowed to heal in. These scars widen. At the knees there is a tendency for seroma collections, which require serial aspirations or a temporary drain.

Cosmetic Abdominoplasty

By far the most common assault to a woman's abdomen is pregnancy.

The cosmetic treatment of the abdomen ranges from simple liposuction to abdominoplasty with muscle repair and umbilical translocation. LipoSelection℠ of the entire abdomen works well if there is no loose skin. Abdominoplasty is the standard approach to improve stomach appearance after aging, pregnancy, and minor fluctuations in weight. The patient desires shapely contours, not just the removal of excess skin.

Many factors affect abdominal contour deformities including localized fat deposits, obesity, muscle and skin laxity, fitness, scars from previous surgery, age, pregnancies, hormone replacement therapy, menopause, and genetics. Between the ages of 45 and 55 many women and men accumulate fat around the abdomen. The upper abdomen in many men and some women cannot be treated by abdominoplasty as the fat is behind the muscle around the organs and not in the subcutaneous tissue.

The most common assault to a woman's abdomen is

pregnancy, especially with large or multiple babies. Not only does the stretched out lower abdominal skin not shrink, but thinning of the abdominal muscles can leave a hernia like protuberance. Both of these problems are reversed by abdominoplasty. The typical patient who undergoes a cosmetic abdominoplasty is quite different in size, shape, and scope from the weight loss surgery patient. However, the aesthetic goals are the same.

When the skin laxity is in only the lower abdomen and liposuction can treat the upper, I recommend a limited abdominoplasty with liposuction. The skin resection is a narrow transverse ellipse of the lower abdomen and the umbilicus is untouched. Some suture tightening of the lower abdominal fascia can be done. For generalized looseness of the abdomen, which is the most common presentation, I perform a complete abdominoplasty, that addresses both loose skin and the central fascial weakness. If there is mild looseness of skin of both the upper and lower abdomen, I employ the latest Brazilian method. In that method skin is removed from both the lower abdomen and the upper, from beneath the breasts. (See photo gallery, page 7)

Let's look at the experience of 33 year old Jill, who exercises vigorously every day. Thin with loose skin she seeks an improved contour and youthful appearance. Prior intra abdominal operations had left her abdomen protuberant with a scallop-like drape of skin. She also hated her thigh saddlebags. All contour deformity was corrected by a circumferential abdominoplasty with a lower body lift.

Jill's Story

"While fairly well-read /studied on all of these counts, I honestly never thought of myself as a serious candidate for elective surgery: in the end, the overwhelming day-to-day unhappiness with my body – despite a hardcore work-out ethic and small pre-surgery size –

*overrode what I formerly considered a needless vanity. But the sig-
nificant scar and tissue from carrying and removing huge fibroids
("nearly the size of a basketball") was also beginning to erode my
self-confidence across the board. I'm told I have a ways to go to full
recovery, but I'm already feeling and looking so much better."*

Extended Panniculectomy

Panniculectomy has a role in the weight loss patient. A panniculectomy is the removal of symptomatic hanging abdominal
skin and fat. If there are medical indications such as recurrent skin
infections or back pain, the costs may be covered by insurance. In
its simplest form a low abdominal transverse segment of skin and
fat is removed and the wound is closed directly without undermining. Unfortunately upper and lateral abdominal bulging will be
emphasized following that limited procedure. If I remove a second
midline vertical ellipse of skin and fat those problems will be ame-
liorated, but at the cost of a long mid line vertical scar. I call that
inverted T shape excision an extended panniculectomy. If there is
already a midline scar or the patient wants optimal improvement
with the least intervention than the extended panniculectomy
should be considered as an effective compromise procedure. For
further description and photographs see Hurwitz D.J. Invited
Discussion of Circular Belt Lipectomy: A retrospective follow up
study on complications and cosmetic result by Huizum, Roche,
Hoffer in *Annals of Plast. Surg.* in press for 2005.

Buttock Augmentation with Fat or Implants

Increasingly patients are asking for enlargement and more
youthful contour of their buttocks. Sometimes the buttocks sag

because of massive weight loss or overzealous liposuction. The once prominent and curvaceous buttock is flat, deflated, and wrinkled. If that is a problem, I pull down some of the low back and upper buttock adipose excess of the lower body lift for auto augmentation of the mid and lower buttocks. The top layer of skin is removed and this mound is slid under the upwardly advanced lower buttock skin flap.

If buttock auto augmentation was not done or leaves inadequate fill, then I offer the options of fat fill by lipoaugmentation or silicone buttock implant augmentation. Lipoaugmentaton is the process of gently aspirating unwanted fat and reinserting it into the body by injection. I achieve success in fat augmentation by placing less than .5 cc's during withdrawal of each plunge of the small cannula. Since each buttock needs around 300 cc's of fat, I must thrust the cannula more than 600 times. Obviously, there must be enough fat available for grafting. Much of the fat is removed from nearby lower back, flanks, and thighs for recess around the buttocks.

When there is not enough fat available, I often use soft silicone elastomer implants. These are rubber like pads roughly the size of dessert plates. They are positioned directly over the gluteus maximus muscles through an incision over the sacrum. Symmetrical placement and maintenance of implant position are concerns.

Lower Leg Deformity

The aesthetic deformity between the knees and ankles ranges from excess skin and fat to being too thin. On the rare occasion that I remove excess skin and fat from this area, I stage a procedure separate from the inner thighplasty. A single operation down the leg may be too risky for deep vein thrombosis. A conservative elliptical excision of medial thigh skin with some liposuction leaves a shapely calf with a fine long scar along the inner back part. For others, who object to marked lower leg thinness, I insert a flounder shaped silicone rubber behind the calf muscles through a short incision behind the knee. A shapely calf is constructed without interference with running.

Chapter **6**

Upper Body Reshaping

The mid torso, breasts, and arms are badly misshapen after massive weight loss. Relative to the lower body, fewer plastic surgeons have experience or confidence in treating this region. This chapter presents state of the art treatment.

The breast deformity can be bizarre. Breasts lose fat causing flattening and poor projection. The glands are floppy. The nipples are distorted and droopy. The breasts may resemble pancakes. These breasts are difficult to reshape. For milder cases silicone implant augmentation with breast reshaping solves the problem. The more severely deformed breasts are reshaped with a mastopexy and nearby flaps.

Compounding the breast problem is the surrounding loose skin of the arm, axilla, chest, and upper abdomen. For some this complex deformity is less tolerable than the lower body disorder. For the majority of weight loss patients, I have been able to mobilize unwanted upper body excess skin and tissue to augment the breasts successfully. Most patients are overwhelmingly pleased with this procedure and delighted to avoid some of the risks associated with breast implants. I have designed an effective and safe approach to simultaneously contour the breast, upper torso, and upper arms called the upper body lift. First, I will discuss the commonly performed breast augmentation and mastopexy

Breast Augmentation and Mastopexy

Breast augmentation and mastopexy (breast lift) may be performed independently or together. Later I will discuss the more complicated interplay of breast reshaping during an upper body lift.

Conceptually, breast enlargement is a straightforward procedure. An FDA (Federal Drug Administration) approved saline filled silicone shelled implant is placed behind the breast. In reality, aesthetic breast augmentation requires artistry, skill and precision. Aesthetic success depends on patient selection, implant selection, my skill and your healing. The ideal patient wants to enlarge a small but attractive breast. Unusually shaped and poorly developed breasts will be larger but not necessarily more attractive after simple augmentation. Additional procedures, such as mastopexy or release of restricting tissues, may be needed.

An implant should augment a breast not overwhelm it. If the volume of the implant is so large that its diameter exceeds that of the breast, then the imperfections of the implant, edges and rippling, will be apparent. Implants today are offered in a variety of shapes and projections for surgeons to select the optimum fit. While much attention is directed toward the location of incision, more important is my skill for a speedy recovery and optimum breast to implant relationships. While I will use the incision that the patient prefers, the one and one-half inch inframammary approach is ideal for precise submuscular placement. Recovery is usually within weeks.

Healing has immense impact on the result. Some patients form tight capsules around the implants leaving a rounded and firm result. This is blunted somewhat by an under the muscle (sub pectoral) approach. Hematoma (blood collection) or minor infections may leave hard capsules. Some patients form too soft capsule, which can lead to visible rippling. If the implant is very large the entire breast sags due to a lack of supporting capsule or surgical violation of the inframammary fold.

I prefer to perform breast augmentation as an outpatient procedure under general anesthesia. For thin patients, I place the implant under the pectoralis muscle. General anesthesia paralyzes the muscle avoiding painful spasms and bleeding. The operation consists of making an incision and then creating a precise pocket for the implant behind the breast. The deflated implant is inserted into the pocket and filled with sterile saline through an infusion set. I prefer an incision in the crease below the breast, but it can also be made around the areola, under the armpit, or concomitant to an abdominoplasty incision.

In the sub pectoral position, the implant is less obvious, softer and smoother. Interpretation of mammography may be easier. In fuller sized women, I am placing the implants under the fascia of the pectoralis muscle and obtaining similar benefits. In that position there can be no unnatural displacement and distortion seen with forceful use of the arms.

At the time of this writing, the FDA permits only saline-filled implants for cosmetic augmentation. The difficulty in diagnosing broken implants and the uncertainty of treating this problem prompts procrastination of general approval. We are hopeful that the high cohesive gel implant will reach the United States market in 2005 because it does not disperse through the tissues when broken. Unfortunately that implant is firmer to the touch than the less cohesive (sticky) implants. While it is unusual to seep through the tissue, I have on occasion removed broken regular gel filled implants. The immediate deflation of saline implants makes breakage obvious and replacement is rather simple for the surgeon and easy on the patient. There is no sci-entific evidence that silicone gel filled implants cause health problems, but some public uncertainty remains. Saline implants are less controversial.

Skin quality and the amount of breast tissue factor into the ultimate decisions surrounding the best procedure for you. Recently saline filled implants have been offered in a variety of profiles. The narrow based high profile implant is especially useful for narrow chested women. Many women are very pleased with medium profile smooth round implants, which are less expensive than teardrop shaped. Some plastic surgeons strongly prefer anatomical shaped implants. The tear drop shape tends to minimize upper breast fullness, which can be advantageous. Anatomical implants must have a textured surface to avoid rotation in their pocket. Textured implants may diminish hardening of the breast by capsular contracture. Unfortunately, they are more likely to develop visible rippling. In the United States, four smooth saline filled implants are implanted for every textured.

Breast Implant Options

Incision:

- Under the breast – inframammary
- Around the nipple areola complex – periareolar
- Under the armpit – transaxillary
- Through the navel – transumbilical
- Through a tummy tuck incision – transabdominoplasty

Implant Surface:

- Textured
- Smooth

Implant Shape:

- Medium, low, and high profile
- Teardrop (anatomical)

Breast implant augmentation does not correct excessive ptosis. A mastopexy is needed. Mastopexy raises and reshapes sagging breasts.

Breasts lose volume after pregnancy and nursing. Along with weight loss, genetic predisposition, and aging, the breasts sag. Some women abhor their unclothed breasts. Mastopexy reshape breasts, creating more youthful perkier appearance. While they usually fade, mastopexy scars are permanent. Accepting the new scars, women tend to be pleased with their breasts after mastopexy. Needing less supportive bras, they are more comfortable with vigorous physical activity wearing leotards and tank tops. This operation also reduces the circumference of the areola, the darker skin around the nipple, which is an important consideration in some. Breast implants inserted during mastopexy improve firmness and volume.

If planning more children, you probably should postpone your breast lift. Breast feeding may be compromised and pregnancy will change your breasts again. The best candidates for mastopexy are healthy, emotionally stable women who have realistic expectations. Ideally, mastopexy candidates should have breasts sized between B and D cup brassieres.

The droopy breast has three distinct problems:

• Loose skin

• Breast tissue too low

• The nipple too low

Mastopexy removes extra skin, reshapes breast tissue, and repositions the nipple.

Mastopexy creates more attractive breasts with additional incisions. More scars are the unavoidable trade off for improved shape. The traditional reduction uses the so-called Wise pattern, leaving an upside down T shaped scar extending from the areola. The long inframammary scar is the most objectionable. In more tubular shaped breasts, the scar can be limited to around the nipple-areola complex. For broader breasts, a short vertical scar from the areola downward may be needed. This vertical limb is added to the mastopexy to project the breast, much like forming a cone from a flat sheet of paper. The removal of skin in a vertical direction allows medial and lateral breast skin to be moved toward the center. This prevents central flattening of the breast sometimes seen in a periareolar mastopexy.

Short scar breast reduction and mastopexy are gaining

acceptance by United States plastic surgeons. The hesitancy is that the immediate result of short scar techniques flattens the lower breast that needs months to mature rounder. Also further excess skin may need to be removed at a second operation. All these short scar techniques eliminate the scar along the inframammary fold. These short scar procedures rely on sutured glandular reshaping to hold shape rather than a smaller but stretchable skin brassiere. The long-term stability of shape is enhanced.

The traditional breast lift has five components:

1 Areola is reduced in size.
2 Breast tissue is repositioned.
3 Nipple and areola are elevated.
4 Extra skin is removed.
5 New skin envelope is fashioned.

One of my patients, Peggy, is pretty typical.
She was just getting through a difficult divorce from a man she had been married to for 12 years. She wanted to do something to make herself feel better. First she thought about having her eyes done, and then she made the mistake of trying on a tight-fitting lycra bodysuit at the mall. "That did it for me. From then on I decided my eyes were good for a few years, and I had to have my breasts done," Peggy told me. She was not prepared for me to recommend a lift along with implants, but after breastfeeding two children, her breasts required increased volume and reshaping which worked well.

Breast augmentation and mastopexy are a difficult combination, because augmentation increases the volume while mastopexy reduces the size of the skin envelope. Scars and areola can be unattractively enlarged. Over time, the lax breast may sag with the weight of the implant. Nevertheless, coincidental breast augmentation with mastopexy with a small to moderate sized implant can yield exceptionally attractive breasts. The problem is more complex in the weight loss patient.

The Weight Loss Upper Deformity

After massive weight loss, breast shape, texture, projection, and skin elasticity are poor. The breasts are displaced and broadened by descended inframammary folds. The nipple areolar complexes are distorted and droopy. Cascading skin rolls of the upper abdomen and mid torso obscure the breasts. Overlapping skin traps moisture with increased bacterial counts and mal odor. Skin irritation leads to skin infections under the breasts and the nearby skin rolls. Bras and undergarments fit poorly.

The upper arms form bat-like wings with hanging skin. The back of the armpit (the posterior axillary fold) descends. The oversized armpit flows into lateral chest rolls. What was once an enticing interplay of alternating convexities and concavities becomes a source of embarrassment. I developed a method to reconstruct this erotic zone of beauty without constricting scars. I call it the L brachioplasty.

Evolution of Upper Body Lift

Until several years ago, I treated the breast deformity in isolation. I ignored the reconstructive potential of nearby skin excess. I came to realize that a circumferential abdominoplasty with a lower body lift, no matter how aggressively pulled, did not adequately correct mid torso laxity. If I moved the belt-like excision closer to the rib cage, the mid torso rolls were reduced, but I lost the improvement on the hips and lateral thighs. Furthermore, patients prefer the hip hugging scars to the waist-high scars. Finally, traditional abdominoplasty, even with more extreme undermining fails to correct loose skin of the upper abdomen. Patients do not like residual upper abdominal skin rolls between the umbilicus and chest.

Coincident with seeking a solution to the breast problem, a better approach to the deformed axilla and upper arm was needed. Leaving behind an oversized axilla, hanging arm skin, and a droopy posterior axillary fold detracted from whatever breast improvement was achieved. An L shaped arm lift was designed that addressed these issues and leaves a curvilinear inner arm scar that zigzags across the axilla to the lateral chest.

To correct the shrunken breast, I at first relied upon silicone implant augmentation, usually with an appropriate mastopexy. Implant augmentation with mastopexy is the accepted method for increasing breast volume and correcting shape. Unfortunately, for the more severe weight loss patient my results sometimes fall short of expectations. In weight loss patients the inelastic skin poorly adapts to the implant. With little parenchyma present, the new breast is dominated by the shape of the implant and its capsule. The capsule is scar responding to the implant. When the capsule thickens and contracts, the breasts are too round and firm. When the capsule is too thin, the implant may descend within the breast like a rock in a sock. Furthermore, the largest implants drift to a low inframammary fold or even beyond. A disturbing bottoming out of the breast with the nipple pointing upward occurs. With weak tissue tensions, the implant ripples. The unnatural depression between the breast and axilla is unaffected by implants. Finally some patients prefer not to accept the risks of silicone implants. They would rather that I use their own tissues, which would otherwise be discarded during a body lift to build up their breasts. The ready availability of this nearby tissue led again to innovation.

Before I discuss my tissue flap augmentation approach, I note that some weight loss patients are suited for an implant augmentation with mastopexy. **(See photo gallery, page 30)** These patients do not have mid torso rolls of skin. They have a distinct, appropriately positioned inframammary fold and reasonable nearby skin contour and laxity. These patients have better breast shape and feel with silicone gel filled implants. One of my patients made the cover of the November 30, 2003 *People Magazine.* (See www.hurwitzcenter.com)

"I owe a huge portion of my confidence to Dr. Hurwitz. People should understand that losing the weight was only part of my battle, a battle that still consisted of my reflection. I was not able to fully become the person I was born to be without his help." – Roberta (Roberta appeared on the Montel Williams Show, Discovery Health Cable, Jane Pauley Show, and People Magazine)

For the overly large but sagging breast, a traditional conservative reduction may be done. **(See photo gallery, page 12)** Their persistent large lower body is best counterbalanced with ample breasts. To improve projection and limit reliance on inelastic skin, I prefer a vertical pattern reduction. However, redundant inelastic skin may require further excision along the inframammary fold. Isolated breast reduction is indicated for patients who desire as few scars as possible or who fail to see the value of an upper body lift. Similarly these patients prefer a standard abdominoplasty to the circumferential scars of a lower body lift. Even when forewarned of their compromise, patients point out their persistent mid torso and hip tissue excess.

An epiphany case taught me that ignoring a descended inframammary fold with loose upper abdominal skin leads to inadequate upper body contouring as well as poor breast aesthetics.

She is a 5' 5", 34 year old who went from 325 to 150 pounds

following gastrointestinal bypass surgery. Her skin just hung on her body with flat and long droopy beasts. I performed a lower body lift, vertical medial thighplasty, and an anchor pattern mastopexy with a 325 cc's saline filled silicone implant augmentation. While her lower body and thighs were greatly improved, she still had mid torso skin laxity. Also her implants bottomed out (went too low). A subsequent reverse abdominoplasty and secondary breast reshaping allowed me to improve her mid torso and better reshape her breasts. Incidentally, eight months later she married for the first time and at the time of this printing, she and her husband are expecting their first child. With her case I learned the importance of the reverse abdominoplasty and establishing a firm inframammary fold. I was on my way to developing the upper body lift. (See photo gallery, page 13)

Upper Body Lift with Breast Reshaping

"The worst part was my arms. That's what I hated the most. The rest of you are always covered. I had to wear long sleeves even in the summer. I felt like I was stuffing my armpit into my bra." – Deborah (See photo gallery, pages 15, 16)

Many of the massive weight loss patients have unsightly mid torso rolls of excess skin, flat drooping breasts, and hanging arm skin that lead into sagging armpits. Five years ago I found no reports of successful treatment of that complex deformity. Independently I designed the upper body portion of Total Body Lift surgery.

The upper body lift is optimally combined with the "L" brachioplasty (arm lift) that extends to the chest, reduces the oversized axilla and raises the droopy posterior axillary fold.

The **four components** to an upper body lift are presented in detail. **Number one** and fundamental is the reverse abdominoplasty, which removes excess skin of the upper abdomen not correctable by standard abdominoplasty. That loose skin is particularly difficult to efface when it is associated with a well-defined roll. The inframammary folds lie on the chest along the bottom of the breasts. These are desirable lines of dermis to muscular fascial adherence which help support and shape the breasts. I estimate the excess skin of the upper abdomen by vigorously pushing upwards and draw a horizontal line from near the sternum to the lateral chest around the mid rib cage. The abdominal skin below the line will be pulled upwards under the breasts. The excess skin above the line will be added to the breasts. The inferiorly based abdominal flaps are undermined below the ribs. A series of strong sutures are placed from this abdominal flap to the sixth rib. While my assistant pushes the flap firmly towards the breasts, I sequentially tied the sutures thereby securing the reverse abdominoplasty flap under the breast, securing a taunt upper abdomen. . Obesity and/or excessive flare of the costal margins make this maneuver difficult.

Component **number two is upward repositioning and securing the descended inframammary fold**. The new inframammary fold position and the reverse abdominoplasty are performed together. With the patient standing, the droopy breast is elevated and the current inframammary folds are sighted and drawn under both breasts. That level is then marked over the sternum. Each breast and inframammary fold is raised to the desired level, which is along the sixth rib and the new inframammary fold position is now registered over the sternum. The procedure is performed as just noted in the last paragraph. The closure of the reverse abdominoplasty forms the inframammary folds and is hidden under the breasts.

Component **number three is correction of the back skin rolls** lateral to and below the breasts. This is planned by pushing excess skin upward on the mid back and lateral chest. When there is appropriate tightening, the horizontal lower incision line is drawn along the bra line. While holding the raised skin in place, the roughly parallel superior incision line is estimated by skin gathering and marked. These two lines continue into the previously marked reverse abdominoplasty lines and lateral limb of the breast reduction pattern. The lines are tapered in the back to close the ellipse near the shoulder blade (scapula). The excision usually runs towards the middle of the back, necessitating removal while the patient is prone. After the back excision is done, the wound is closed in two layers.

Component **number four is reshaping the breasts**. If the breasts have adequate or excess volume, they are reshaped or reduced using an inverted T pattern and central pedicle. If the breasts are small and misshapen, they are difficult to reconstruct with implants and mastopexy. These breasts are shaped and augmented with nearby deepithelialized flaps. In essence, I skin (deepithelialize) excess skin and fat of the mid torso rolls in continuity with the central breast mount. I isolate and rotate around the breast these two flaps. The upper abdominal flap is an inferior extension of the central breast. The lateral flap is a tongue-like lateral flap extension of the central breast. I call these breast building tissue, spiral flaps because they rotate around the breast. **(See breast diagrams in photo gallery, page 17)**

The spiral flaps are created from unwanted excess tissue. These flaps are mobile enough to permit artistic creativity in shaping and augmentation. The breasts are not only enlarged and well shaped, but soft and shift naturally with change in body position. The constricted inferior breast can be beautifully filled. Sensual tapering of the breast into the axilla is possible for the first time.

Optimum and efficient recruitment of nearby soft tissue for breast reshaping requires the just described pre-operative determination of mid torso and upper abdominal excess. With an artistic sense and clinical experience, gather and pinch techniques will faithfully present the excess available for deepithelialized flaps. Planning for the upper body lift begins after the lower lift/abdominoplasty is drawn or previously performed. If a single stage Total Body Lift surgery is planned, then the anticipated inferior torso skin closure tensions are considered.

After all the flaps are prepared, reconstruction begins with suturing the reverse abdominoplasty flap to the sixth rib and thereby, establishing a secure inframammary fold. The excess upper abdominal deepithelialized flap is rolled on itself and sutured to fill out the inferior breast. Then the medially based lateral thoracic flap, also attached to the central breast mound, is turned upward along the lateral chest line. The flap is sutured all the way over toward the sternum near the third rib. The lateral breast contour is set by suturing the dermis of the lateral flap to chest muscle. A tight closure of the lateral thoracic flap donor site from the axilla to the inframammary fold appropriately flattens this area, emphasizes the newly created lateral breast fullness, and improves breast projection. The lateral chest donor site closure is continuous with the advanced and stabilized new inframammary fold. The firm fold also improves breast projection and eliminates bottoming out. (See photo gallery, page 18)

If this soft tissue reconstruction seems too small, I usually stage the silicone implant augmentation for another time. The time consuming and complex tissue resections and rearrangements of the upper body lift as well as the additional devascularization intrinsic to creating a space for the implant makes simultaneous implant and auto augmentation procedures precarious. Moving the nipple upward requires excision of intervening skin, sometimes making the skin closure with precarious flaps over an additional volume of implant too tight.

The upper body lift is complete; however, for most patients the culminating step is my L brachioplasty. I have originated an operation that not only reduces upper arm excess tissue, but also raises the skin fold junction with the axilla, narrows the armpit, and completes the lateral chest shaping. Older techniques ignored the hanging folds and chest excess. Prior techniques also left unnatural T shaped flaps in the axilla that was vulnerable to skin necrosis and thicken scars.

I excise excess skin and fat in the form of an inverted "L" with the long limb along the inner aspect of the upper arm, the short limb across the axilla, and down the chest. The closed angle lies across the dome of the axilla. With healing, the final scar courses along the inferior medial arm, rises to the axillary dome, and then drops vertically to the chest, forming an inverted L.

I close the arm and chest wounds with two layers of absorbable sutures, so that no sutures have to be removed later. I cover the chest and breast closures in gauze, and apply a surgical bra and elastic sleeves. No constricting binder is place across the mid abdomen. Patients are admitted for a single night's observation and care.

The upper body lift is often the second stage operation of Total Body Lift surgery. For most patients, these complex procedures about the breasts are secondary to the lower body reconstruction. Other patients are more concerned about their breast and arm deformity. Then I operate there first. My preference is to start with the abdominoplasty and lower body lift. It is the more traumatic session and takes a longer convalescence. When they are satisfied with the lower body lift, I have their trust and can proceed with the less traumatic upper body lift. We use the second operative session to touch up contours or scars from the first.

The new L shaped arm lift compliments the upper body lift by reducing the axilla, correcting posterior axillary fold ptosis, and further reducing lateral chest rolls. When not performed in tandem, the aesthetic improvement of the breasts is diminished. While plastic surgeons have paid little attention to the beauty and sensuality of the female breast, axilla, and upper arm interplay, it has not been lost in evening fashion, entertainment, and art. Fortunately, the scar does not restrict outstretched arms.

The cutaneous axilla (armpit) is a dome shaped structure formed by the tight adherence of thin axillary skin to deep suspensory fascia. Unseen with the arms at the side, the armpit crevasse is seductively deepest when the arm is extend 90 degrees and gently undulating with the arm fully raised. The L brachioplasty restores these anatomical subtleties in both the weight loss and aging patient without an obtrusive scar. The success is due to the rather large resection of skin and the direct triangular flap advancement of the posterior axillary fold. There are no geometric scars or dog ears due to Z plasties.

In recent years, I have used this L shaped arm lift technique along with the upper body lift for my massive weight loss patients. Ultrasonic assisted lipoplasty may be used to further reduce the size of the arms in patients with excess fat. Our patients can happily wear sleeveless tops as their inner arm scars are not visible during most positions. I have also successfully applied this technique without an upper body lift to non-weight loss aging patients.

Informed consent is a process of physician and staff education. At the initial consultation I introduce the upper body lift and breast reshaping. The patient learns that this is a new procedure, which has considerable merit over prior techniques. As in any operation, but especially due to limited experience and complexity, problems may occur. If recognized these may be treated at the initial procedure or revision surgery including silicone implant insertion may be appropriate. Alternative and more conservative approaches are explained.

Carlene's Story (see photo gallery)

Like so many of my patients, Carlene's weight struggles were a lifelong problem for her. At her largest, she tipped the scales at 320 pounds. As soon as she heard about gastric bypass, she decided she had to do it. She followed Carnie Wilson's saga and expected that she would need plastic surgery afterwards. As a municipal employee, and a divorced mother of a teenage son, Carlene mortgaged her house for twice what she paid and took money out of her retirement fund to finance her surgical reincarnation. The first stage entailed an upper body lift to address her back rolls and waist. That procedure took nine hours. The second operation took 11 hours. It involved a breast reduction, arm lift, and vertical thighplasty, as well as a full facelift. As Carlene says, "I looked at myself in the mirror, and I knew that if I didn't do my neck too I would be sorry." After her breast reduction procedure, she told me that it was the first time since puberty that she didn't have to wear a support bra. She is now a comfortable 38C. Since her gastric bypass surgery, she has lost half her body weight, and has gone through three wardrobes. "In the past, all I ever wore were white running shoes. Now I own 75 pairs of designer shoes," says Carlene.

Of all the components of body contouring, I find the upper body lift and flap breast reshaping extraordinary. What keeps me enthusiastic throughout these exhausting procedures is the confidence that the result will be dramatic and appreciated. Breast reshaping is integral to Total Body Lift surgery. Tissues that would normally be discarded during a reverse abdominoplasty and back roll excision can be very useful. The time flies as I coordinate team surgery.

Jane's Story

"2004 was going to be my year. A year in which I took control of how I wanted to look. I was 55 years old, post menopausal, have dieted and exercised most of my life. I just retired from a profession that I was weighed for the first 14 years of it. So how I looked and felt about myself has always been an issue for me. For the past few years no matter how much I exercised or watched what I ate I could not change my breast and hip size. These two areas have always been a problem for me. With being older the size of my breasts seemed to be heavier and a pain in my back. As far back as I can remember my hips always had fatty deposits sitting on top of them I had thought about and talked about breast reduction but the surgery and the scarring scared me. So at the height of my disgust I called Dr. Hurwitz's office to schedule an appointment. At the first meeting we discussed breast reduction and liposuction for my hip area. He agreed that my breasts were very large and a candidate for reduction and my hip area could be greatly helped with the liposuction. We also discussed liposuction in my midriff area, back, and stomach. Because he felt the skin would be loose in the stomach area we decided on a limited abdominoplasty. My surgery was scheduled and to say I was not scared would be a lie. My greatest supporter was my husband. He loved my body just the way it was but knew how unhappy I had been. I was a DD and hoped to become a C. The morning of the surgery Dr. Hurwitz and his team came to my room and proceeded to prepare me for surgery. He drew all over my breasts and the other areas. He then took pictures.

"When I awoke in recovery I was glad to be staying overnight. I cannot lie. I was very, very uncomfortable. I had given myself ten days to rest and recover. It was painful to lie down, get up, sleep, and do anything. The pain medication helped as I wanted to sleep and be out of the discomfort. The staff was wonderful assuring me that it all was normal. Dr. Hurwitz explained that with the

incisions and the swelling made everything so tight. He said the swelling would go down over the next three months. I really did not believe him. I had the surgery on Monday and by Friday my husband came home from work to find me crying. I felt I had made the biggest mistake of my life.

"After five weeks I was permitted to go back to exercising and to play golf. I have to admit at that time I liked how my breasts looked in clothes. I tried jackets and tops on that I had not worn in a few years. It was great. I went to a party and wore a dress without a bra as it had thin straps. It was wonderful. I have to admit the other parts of my body were looking good too and even better in clothes. The best part is that my husband was thrilled. He loves how I look, and so do I. Well it is now eight weeks since the surgery. I can see that the swelling is going down and things do feel better. Imagine that. I love how I feel about myself now and especially not having the discomfort of the large breasts. I thought about the surgery and realize it's a bit like being pregnant. The pain was terrible while you are going through it but than you forget how bad it was. Your reward is a body that looks better on you." (See photo gallery, Mary page 7)

Brachioplasty for the Aging Rachioplasty Patient

Upper arm fat, flabbiness, and loose hanging skin commonly cause embarrassment. Women avoid wearing sleeveless clothing even on the hottest summer days. Increasingly women are choosing cosmetic plastic surgery to reduce their upper arms. Before recent improvements in liposuction and technique, I discouraged surgery for mild to moderate deformity. As aesthetic surgeons, our goal is always to provide a result in which the operation is as undetectable as possible. When there is hanging skin, upper arm reduction leaves an uncovered scar.

Today, women with excess upper arm fat but good skin tone can have contour improvement with liposuction alone, leaving tiny incisions. Small diameter long cannulae are used to minimize connective tissue trauma. I prefer the preliminary use of ultrasound, usually the Vaser®, which leaves the least damage and best tightening. Month long sleeve compression aids in skin retraction.

However, for patients requiring more extensive surgery, my L brachioplasty incision usually begins in the armpit area, called the axilla, and runs along the underside of the arm and down the chest in the form of an L. The incisions are made toward the back so that the scar is not visible with the arms in their normal resting position. Over time, the scars are thinner, softer, and less noticeable.

"The worst part was my arms. That's what I hated the most. The rest of you is always covered. I had to wear long sleeves even in the summer. I felt like I was stuffing my armpit into my bra." – Deborah (See photo gallery, pages 15, 16)

Chapter 7

Total Body Lift™ Surgery for Men Only

In this chapter men finally get their due. So far I have written this book from the feminine perspective. Much of the information transfers to men, but there are important differences. Males want to be rid of their sagging breasts. Their love handles around the flanks can be enormous. Their upper abdominal girth is often prominent. While the hips and outer thighs do not sag as much as in women, the inner thighs often have hanging rolls. Loose skin of the upper arms is rarely a problem. We continue with a detailed discussion of the enlarged male breasts called gynecomastia.

Gynecomastia (Male Breast enlargement)

Male breast enlargement called gynecomastia is common. Often appearing in adolescence, it affects nearly 40 percent of men at one time or another. Gynecomastia is a combination of dense breast glandular tissue behind the nipple that mixes with adipose as it fans out over the pectoralis major muscle. It may be unilateral (one side) or bilateral (both sides). The male breast appears fuller and rounded compared with the ideal flattened and rectangular male anterior chest contour. In pseudo gynecomastia, breast enlargement is principally the result of excess fat accumulation. True gynecomastia is a proliferation of the glandular breast parenchyma with some minor increase in adipose.

Gynecomastia can be the enlargement of the normal male breast bud due to circulating estrogens. Abnormal sources of excessive estrogen output must be considered and the list of serious medical conditions causing that is on the opposite page.

The surgeon considers all these causes. If none are present, as is usually the situation, then the etiology is referred to as idiopathic. Idiopathic means we do not exactly know the reason for the enlargement. We believe the gynecomastia is due to heightened sensitivity to the normal circulation of small

Underlying Causes of Gynecomastia

Drug-Induced

- Antiretroviral therapy
- Androgenic steroids
- Spironolactone
- Anti acid therapy
- Anti cancer drugs
- Oral contraceptives
- Digitalis
- Marijuana, heroin
- Estrogens

Estrogen-Testosterone Imbalance

- Increased estrogen secretion states
- Male and female genetic make up
- Genetic disorder
- Congenital adrenal hyperplasia

Increased Peripheral Conversion to Estrogen

- Adrenal disease
- Liver disease
- Excess thyroid hormone

Neoplasm

- Testicular tumors
- Adrenal tumors
- Hormone-producing neoplasms
- Reduced testosterone production or activation

amounts of estrogen and estrogen like products from the adrenals and testicles. As men age or suffer from obesity, testosterone deficiency relative to normal estrogens is the source of breast stimulation.

The typical patient has fullness in his chest and breast area. This is usually fat but may also be some of the residual breast gland noted by firmness just below the nipple. The fat or fullness may extend around the side to the edge of the pectoralis muscle and into the armpits. The patient may desire a flatter, more defined breast and chest shape, and/or flatter and smaller nipples and areolae (pigmented areas of the nipple).

Men may be embarrassed and extremely self-conscious about their feminized appearing breasts. When dealing with adolescents, the psychological burden can lead to social isolation. Concerned parents sometimes report their sons withdraw from peers to avoid the gym or visits to the beach, summer camp, or other outdoor activities. Let us look at the example of my patient Henry, who suffered with gynecomastia throughout his adolescence and into adulthood.

Henry's Story

"Summers were the worst for me. We lived at the shore and going to the beach was out of the question. I was the only guy on my block who would not be seen without a tee shirt on in August. When I was growing up, cosmetic surgery wasn't something anyone discussed in my family. I had to wait until I was out on my own to have it done. Making the first consultation was the hardest part. The idea of having to get naked in front of the doctor and his nurse caused me to break out into a cold sweat. But after I got comfortable with Dr. Hurwitz' staff, the whole thing seemed simple, like why hadn't I done this sooner. Even the operation was not too bad. I focused on the outcome and the discomfort was minor. People have commented that my personality has totally

changed after the surgery. They feel that I am much more open and that my new self-confidence shines through. I know that I am smiling more at people and they are smiling back, and women respond totally different to me. I feel so proud of my accomplishment and glad I had the courage to undertake this surgery. For any of you guys out there who have the same problem as I did, just do it."

A complete physical exam is performed, looking for possible secondary causes, such as obesity, liver enlargement, or testicular tumors. Palpation of the breast determines the predominant tissues. Glandular tissue is firm, almost gritty. Fat is soft. The volume and shape of the breast deformity as well as the quality of the overlying skin is assessed. Nipple areolar complex malposition and enlargement are quantified.

Middle aged and older men need routine pre-operative tests, such as chest x-ray, blood count, liver function studies, urine analysis, and electrocardiogram. At any age, if the history or physical exam implies a possible underlying medical problem, consultation with appropriate medical specialists, including an endocrinologist is arranged. Medications and drugs that may stimulate breast glands are stopped, followed by a period of observation. I request obese patients to lose weight. Unless the deformity is severe, I delay operations until maturity for teenagers because the gynecomastia is likely to regress. If there is no resolution of the gynecomastia, the only effective treatment is surgery.

In general, in adolescents with visible breast enlargement, there is a glandular type or combination of glandular-adipose. Middle-aged and elderly men have a tendency to accumulate more adipose. Older men tend to have adipose exclusively.

Gynecomastia is a fairly common cosmetic problem, with significant psychological overlay. Surgery varies according to the

For guiding treatment, Jerome Webster classified gynecomastia by quality of tissues.

1 glandular only

2 fatty glandular mixed

3 simple fatty

In 1973 Simon, Hoffman and Kahn categorized gynecomastia by size.

I minor but visible breast enlargement, no skin redundancy

II moderate breast enlargement; no skin redundancy

III moderate breast enlargement; with minor skin redundancy

IV gross breast enlargement, severe skin redundancy

deformity. Since the aesthetic outcome is the issue, excessive scarring and contour irregularities should be avoided. The common trans-areolar approach is cosmetically appealing since the scar does not extend to surrounding skin.

I usually use a combination approach of tumescent infiltration, ultrasonic assisted lipoplasty (UAL) and then liposuction. If there is residual gland I remove most of it by sharp dissection through an intra-areolar incision. This approach provides very satisfactory, aesthetically pleasing results for patients with glandular and mixed gynecomastia (Webster I and II). Webster III gynecomastia patients reap the greatest benefits from UAL and liposuction, because that may induce significant skin reduction due to retention of bridging fibroelastic tissue. LipoSelection℠ by Vaser® appears best at that.

I initiate most gynecomastia operations with UAL followed by suction. There is considerably less bleeding. There is minimal swelling and no post-operative hematomas with that treatment because of the retention of vascular and connective tissue attachments to the skin. With liposuction over a broad area of the chest, I am able to obtain smoother contours and better skin retraction, avoiding large skin resection except for class IV cases. **(See photo gallery, page 20)**

Massive weight loss men generally present with Class IV deformity. A skin resection leaves a long scar that cannot be hidden on a male chest. Plastic surgeons struggle to leave the least conspicuous scar. I would rather leave a small amount of skin excess than create a long scar. If the skin excess is minimal then I remove it by a doughnut ring like excision around the areola. That leaves a scar only around the areola with radiating folds of skin due to a larger outside ring of skin close to a smaller inside ring. Unfortunately these folds will not smooth out over time in the weight loss patient, because the skin has lost its elasticity. A common technique is to remove the ptotic nipple. The gynecomastia is cut out along a long horizontal ellipse. Then the excised nipple is grafted onto the chest in the proper location. However, the nipple graft often looks unnatural and a long straight scar is conspicuous.

I designed a new operation for the treatment of severe gynecomastia in the weight loss patient and published a case in the Annals of Plastic Surgery in May 2004. I have done many since. This operation considers biomechanical and aesthetic issues. Since the skin excess is both transverse and horizontal, I remove it and the gynecomastia through two obliquely oriented long ellipses of skin and breast tissue that drape around the nipple. That leaves behind a triangular flap to support the nipple. That triangular base flap has excess fat and breast. I reduce it with UAL, along with disruption of the inframammary fold. The resulting scar has a short limb that starts near the lower sternum, rises to arch the areola and then descends toward the lower outer chest. Since the areola seems to break up the scar, it appears as if it were two smaller scars. The scar that wraps around the areola is less conspicuous than a straight line scar. The excision pattern resembles a boomerang, so I call this operation the boomerang gynecomastia correction. In some cases further reduction of the base was necessary at a later procedure. The ideal patient has a hairy chest, which hides the scar. **(See photo gallery, page 21)**

"Physically life is grand. I have so much more energy to work and to play. I am not burdened with the constant pain that was crippling me. Now I can be as active as I have time for. I feel like I have to make up for many wasted years." – Andrew

Chapter **8**

Getting Ready for Surgery

In Chapter Three, I presented the initial body contouring consultation in detail. Before embarking upon major surgery, my patients have multiple opportunities to discuss related issues. When there is an intense desire, I know the patient accepts the risks, prolonged recovery, and expense. Accurate information portrayed in a caring manner relieves anxiety. Some candidates request to speak to others who have gone through similar procedures. I have many patients who have volunteered to share their experiences.

"I got into a size 8! Low cut! I can't believe it!" – *Alicia*

"I am so much happier now. I really feel that I have reaped all the benefits of the changes I made." – *Donna*

Deborah's Story (see photo gallery)

Deborah had Total Body Lift surgery December 22, 2003 and was discharged on Christmas Eve. Her story and surgery was televised on WTAE evening news, Pittsburgh's ABC affiliate. She was part of a two part series produced by medical editor Marilyn Brooks. With her incredible transformation, Deborah is one of my biggest fans. When she came to see me, she was eager to salvage the tattoo of a yin yang symbol that she got to camouflage a spider bite on her left hip. We were able to save the tattoo, but ended up moving it to her back right above the buttocks crease. After her operations, she went from a size 26 to svelte size 6 dress. She went back to the firm she worked at for six years, and no one recognized her. Her greatest joy in life is to go to places where people used to know her at 306 pounds and have no idea who she is until she opens her mouth or gives them her name. For Deborah, my surgery was like giving herself a big present. As she says, "It's like my new truck only it lasts much longer."

Susan's Story

"Most of my life my prayers were for weight loss and a healthy decent body. I do know God answers our prayers and gives us our desires. He led me to you. I never expected the wonderful results or a body as beautiful as you have created for me. I used to avoid mirrors and now I really like who I see. God has given you a brilliant mind and you are truly an artist. So dear Dr. Hurwitz for all of this I am thanking you. You have changed my life forever. Thank you!"

Pre-Operative Photography

Patient photographs are for the plastic surgeon what x-rays are for orthopedic surgeons.

Patient photography is essential to planning. Posing is awkward to the patient, but they are pleased to have them for later comparison. Placing her in standardized positions gives me an opportunity to look for subtleties through the calibrating camera lens. Patient photographs are for the plastic surgeon what x-rays are for orthopedic surgeons. They assist in defining the deformity and operative planning. I take the color copies to the pre-operative marking area to confirm their accuracy. Due to archiving errors, lighting, skewed positioning, short focal length, change in patient's weight, pictures can unintentionally mislead. Those confirmed photos with attached notes hang in the operating room, reminding me of the deformity while standing. With permission these photographs help me teach others.

For Smokers Only

While every adult realizes that smoking is unhealthy, it has unique adverse consequences during plastic surgery. Smoking causes constriction (narrowing) of small blood vessels in the skin, which adversely effects healing. Skin movement requires undermining prior to use for reconstruction. The process of undercutting skin partially devascularizes it. Tense closure and swelling also reduces nutrient blood flow. Then you add nicotine from cigarette smoke and skin circulation is even further reduced. At some point of diminished skin circulation vitality is lost. The skin flap margin turns blue then black and dies. Nearby is ischemic (poor blood flow) skin and fat, which is susceptible to infection, and spreads the skin necrosis and endangers the patient. When massive undermined flaps are involved, the consequences could be lethal.

For those reasons I do not knowingly perform major body contouring surgery on smokers. If you have had successful abdominoplasty in the past while smoking consider yourself lucky. Smokers must stop one month prior to scheduled major body contouring surgery, and not resume until one month later.

Medications to Avoid Before Surgery

Prior to surgery, you need to discontinue certain prescription medications, over-the-counter medications, and vitamins. Take no more aspirin or vitamin E capsules for two weeks prior. Aspirin, nonsteroidal anti-inflammatory medications (e.g.: ibuprofen), and vitamin E can cause excessive bleeding. Medications categorized

Suggested Medications to Avoid Pre-Operation

Advil	Doan's	Percodan-Demi
Aleve	Dolia	Persantine
Alka-Seltzer	Dolobid	Persistin
Anacin	Dristan	Quagesic
Anaprox	Duradyne	Relafen
Anaproxn	Duragesic	Robaxisal
Ansaid	Easprin	Rufen
APC	Ecotrin	Sine-aid
Arthritis Pain Formula	Empirin	Sine-off
ASA	Emprazil	Soma with Codeine
Ascriptin	Equagesic	Soma Compound
Ascodeen-30	Excedrin	Stanback Powder
Aspercream	Feldene	Max Powder
Aspergum	Fiorinal	Stendin
Aspirin	Flurbiprophen Sodium	Stero-Darvon w/ASA
Bayer Aspirin	Four Way Cold	Supac
BC Cold Powder	Goody's Extra Strength	SX-65 compound
BC Powders	Ibuprofen	Synalgos
Brufen	Indocin	Synalgos DC
Buff-A-Corn	Indomethacin	Talwin
Buffadyne	Magsal	Tolectin
Bufferin	Measurin	Toradol
Buffex	Meclomen	Trandate
Butalbital	Medipren	Trental
Cama Arthritis Pain Reliever	Midol-200	Trialgesic
Cama-Inlay	Midol	Triaminicin
Caprin	Midol PMS	Trilisate
Caspirin	Mobigesic	Ursinus Inlay
Cephalgesic	Monacet with codeine	Vanquish
Cheracol	Momentum Muscle Back Form	Vivo Med
Children's Aspirin	Motrin	Vitaman E
Clinoril	Naprosyn	Voltaren
Conaterol	Norgesic	Wesprin
Congespirin	Norgesic Forte	Zactrin
Cope	Nuprin	Zorpin
Coricidin	Pabirin buffered	Gingko
Coumadin	Panadynes	Rogaine
Darvon with ASA	Panalgesic	Pepto-Bismol
Darvon Compound	Daypro	
Disalcid	Percodan	

as monoamine oxidase (MAO) inhibitors (e.g., the antidepressants
Nardil or Parnate) are contraindicated because of their adverse
interactions with narcotics and vasoconstrictors. Also avoid
alcoholic beverages which depress mentation and liver function.

Herbal and Dietary Supplements

An estimated 60 million people in the United States self medicate with herbal remedies. For many, the words "natural," herbal," or "alternative medicine conjure up images of safety and purity. Unfortunately, this inaccurate perception creates a false sense of security.

Botanicals (products made from plant life such as roots, barks, or herbs), as well as vitamin and mineral supplements are chemically active substances that can have powerful effects on the body. Willow bark, for example, was used over 1,000 years ago to reduce fever and pain. The active ingredient in willow bark, salicin, is a predecessor of a class of drugs called salicylates. Aspirin is a salicylate and as already mentioned that drug causes poor clotting.

Like pharmaceutical medications, herbal remedies and dietary supplements can cause adverse effects and interact unpredictably with other prescription medications. There are a growing number of alarming reports from doctors' offices and medical centers around the country, some of which have been filed with the Food and Drug Administration's (FDA) MedWatch program.

Herbal ingredients such as chaparral, comfrey, and ephedra (Ma huang), Vitamins A, B6, niacin, and L-tryptophan (an amino acid), have been cited as health hazards. The FDA warns against using "plantain" because it contains components of the plant Digitalis lanata, which can cause fatal heart reactions.

FDA Regulation

Unlike prescription or even over-the-counter medications, dietary supplements are introduced without the FDA's approval for safety and effectiveness. For the FDA to be able to remove a supplement from the market, it must recognize it is as unsafe only after adverse events are reported. The Federal Trade Commission (FTC) continues to issue better guidelines for the marketing of supplements.

When patients do not disclose their herbal supplements, because they believe these supplements "do not count," unexpected drug interactions may occur. St. John's Wort, an herb with purported effects on mood and sleep disorders, behaves like an MAO inhibitor. Gingko biloba, which comes from the Chinese maidenhair tree and is commonly claimed to enhance memory, has anticoagulation effects more potent that vitamin E. Melatonin, used to induce sleep, may compound the effect of the anesthesia. Echinacea, used to stimulate the immune system, can cause liver damage and blood pressure abnormalities.

My staff and I are convinced that Arnica from the flower Arnica Montana and Bromelain, an enzyme from pineapples, decreases post-operative bruising and swelling. To ensure proper dosage and quality, I give my patients their perioperative supply.

Skin Care

Massive weight loss may lead to chronic minor skin infections between rubbing flaps of skin. These should be taken care of with proper hygiene and drying techniques. If unable to achieve complete improvement, the operation will be limited.

For facial operations, we have considerable experience in skin conditioning. Dry skin is moisturized and oily skin is dried. Glycolic acids, Retin A®, and microdermabrasion are expertly combined. Intense pulsed light and Yag lasers are used to improve pigmentation, remove vascular lesions, and reduce wrinkles. The same rules apply to the skin of the body but to a limited degree.

Presurgical Endermologie® treatments often help skin to contract after liposuction.

Diet & Fitness

As discussed in Chapter Two, body contouring patients should not be obese. Furthermore weight loss should have been stable for four months. If considerable weight loss continues after contouring surgery, then new skin laxity and disappointment will occur. Weight gain after contouring surgery is also disappointing, because some of the contour improvement will be lost.

Some intestinal bypass patients are protein deficient. I have to anticipate and unravel that problem before surgery. Malnutrition can result from a variety of medical problems. Gastric inlet restriction can cause recurrent vomiting. Dietary sensitivities or aversions lead to nutritional deficiencies. Excessive intestinal bypass causes chronic diarrhea, fatty stools, and malabsorption of vital nutrients. Blood tests detect anemia, low serum proteins, and liver dysfunction. I have a certified nutritionist that assists my patients with a healthy diet.

Overweight patients are acceptable candidates for plastic surgery. But if you are obese (BMI over 30), I will ask you to lose some weight. In 2004 I initiated the A.W. Simeon weight loss method, which I discussed in Chapter Three. Many patients who have hit the wall with weight loss attempts have under the direction of my nutritionist, safely shed 20 to 30 pounds over a 40 day course of 500 calorie diet and HCG hormone.

Physical fitness is another important matter. Lengthy operations should be considered a marathon, best performed on well-conditioned patients. So I encourage increasing aerobic exercise in the months prior to surgery. I operate on couch potatoes, but recovery is quicker for those in good health.

"The instructors encouraged me and were a key to my success. Men in the gym recognized me as a human being." – Laura

---

"I lost 150 pounds, and under these clothes I look like a Sharpei puppy. When Dr. Hurwitz asked me what areas I wanted to improve, I didn't know where to begin!" – Maria (See photo gallery, pages 3 to 5)

Chapter 9

Early Recovery Program

With experience gained over nearly three decades of practice, I have helped organize an optimum care environment and team of talented, dedicated surgeons, nurses, coordinators, physician assistants, and a nutritionist. My stylish penthouse office suite at the entrance of the Oakland section of Pittsburgh (home of the University of Pittsburgh Medical Center), is an inviting destination locally or from our nearby international airport. My patients are treated in a highly ranked nationally recognized tertiary care hospital, Magee Women's Hospital of the University of Pittsburgh Medical Center. While fully equipped to handle all medical contingencies, Magee Women's caters to the most discerning cosmetic patient. The hospital has organized a center of excellence for the care of cosmetic and bariatric patients. We have high quality and reasonably priced short stay care. The hospital is surrounded by hotels. The plastic surgery residents, who assist in surgery and hospital care, are among the best in the country. With constant surveillance, we are likely to preempt problems before they become serious.

Good Post-Operative Management

After your body lift, you awake from anesthesia in the operating room, not fully oriented. Later in the recovery room I will apprise you of the results. It will be hard for you to focus, but as I guide your hand over your new contours you should be delighted. That mass of hanging, flopping tissue is gone, replaced by a shape you may have only dreamed of up until now.

Your immediate pain is diminished by the residual effect of the large dose of local anesthetic in your tissues. Later in the day as the numbing medicine wears off you can begin intravenous self administration of small doses of narcotics. Some patients are relieved about how little pain they suffer. Others find the first week's recovery miserable. It is more difficult than the recovery following minimally invasive bariatric surgery. Patients agree that the discomfort was worth the results and are pleased that the improvement is rapid.

You will spend the next half day in bed, not interested in moving much. Nurses will encourage you to breath deeply to avoid lung collapse and congestion. Your legs will be continuously massaged by alternating pressure stocking that move static venous blood toward the heart. These are risk free effective means to prevent leg thrombophlebitis and pulmonary embolism. All of your caregivers will be checking the status of your incisions. Minor openings need to be treated within hours with bedside suture closure. Over the hundreds of my operations, that has occurred only a few times. That is surprising considering the high tension placed.

Your three day hospitalization makes you as comfortable as possible, reverses the ill effects of prolonged anesthesia and modulates your response to surgical trauma. Nausea is a common side effect of general anesthesia. Newer medications keep vomiting to a minimum. Your have lost blood during the operation and your blood pressure may drop, despite adequate intravenous fluids. A low blood concentration as measured by your hematocrit leaves you weak and dizzy. If allowed to go too low you may faint when walking, which is dangerous. Transfusions will then be necessary. If your donated blood in your behalf, you will receive that and sometimes more. Pittsburgh is blessed will a well run voluntary blood bank.

Major operations with large incisions are accompanied by a generalized endocrine response and early wound healing inflammation. The normal reaction of the tissues after injury is the secretion of antidiuretic hormones, which means significant fluid retention. Despite the removal of 10 to 20 pounds of flesh, you will actually gain weight due to fluid retention. Some of this water manifests as swelling in the feet and ankles. All healing areas will be inflamed with increased blood flow, resulting in swelling of the operative sites. With body contouring surgery that means a large area of the body. The heavier the tissue, the greater is the effect.

The immediate response of the blood supply to the area is constriction of the vessels. This is followed immediately by vasodilation that allows fluid to exit the capillaries and flood the area. Chemicals in the plasma and on injured tissues attract white blood cells that enter the area and start to clean up foreign material, bacteria, and dead cells.

Drains

Half-inch wide, multiperforated silicone tube drains are placed through the back, along the incisions and down to the outer thighs. These are connected to squeeze bulbs that suck out fluid. Later in the operation two more suction drains are placed under the upper abdominal flap. At first excess infiltration fluid and some blood is removed. Then some weeping serum is evacuated. It takes about two weeks for the drainage to run its course at which time the tubes are removed. A single plastic suture secures the drain in place. After it is cut, the drain is quickly withdrawn, usually with minimal discomfort. Over the next few days, some fluid will leak from the drain site as it spontaneously closes.

Compression Garments

After surgery, my patients wear compression garments contin-uously for the first five days. We normally have patients keep wearing their garments for one month, changing them as needed to offer compression to their newly shrinking size. Most of our patients actually feel better wearing some form of com-pression, which helps to minimize swelling. They are instructed to wear their garment progressively less from week one to week four.

Surgical Guidelines

Procedure	Hospital Discharge	Drains Used	Dressings Off	Sutures Out	Shower
Lipoplasty	Same day	none	5 days	5 days	5 days
Large volume liposuction	Next day	Sometimes	5 days	5 days	5 days
Abdominoplasty	Same day	Two	1 week	dissolve	5 days
Upper Body Lift	Next day	Two	1 week	1 week	5 days
Breast Lift or Reduction	Same day	None	5 days	dissolve	5 days
Breast Augmentation	Same day	None	5 days	1 week	5days
Lower Body Lift	3 days	4 drains	5 days	Dissolve	5 days
Inner Thigh Lift	Same day	None	5 days	Dissolve	5 days
Arm Lift	Same day	None	5 days	Dissolve	5 days
Total Body Lift	3 to 5 days	6 drains	5 days	Dissolve	5 days

Incision Healing

The wound healing process is a complex series of events that
begins at the moment of injury and continues for months to years.
A thin coagulum of fibrin (from the tissues and serum) and red
cells forms a clot that unites the edges of the wound. Eventually
the clot is replaced by granulation tissue, a connective tissue with
a rich blood supply. Scars are red because of increased small
vessels, and the color gradually fades to white as the vascular-

Wound Healing

I - Inflammatory Phase - Immediate to 2 to 5 days

Hemostasis

Vasoconstriction – vessels narrow

Platelet aggregation

Thromboplastin – time it takes blood to clot

Inflammation

Vasodilation – blood flow

Phagocytosis – white cell leaves the blood vessel

II- Proliferative Phase - 2 days to 3 weeks

Granulation

Fibroblasts lay bed of collagen

Fills defect and produces new capillaries

Contraction

Wound edges pull together to reduce defect

Epithelialization

Crosses moist surface

Cell travel 3 cm from point of origin in all directions

III - Remodelling Phase - 3 weeks to 2 years

New collagen forms which increases tensile strength to wounds

Scar tissue is only 80 percent as strong as original tissue

---

ization decreases and the collagen matrix matures. Remodeling of the collagen matrix may continue for years depending on individual genetics and age. In general a thin pale long scar remains when the scars are mature.

Many variables can affect the severity of scarring, including the size and depth of the wound, the blood supply to the area, the thickness and color of your skin, and the direction of the scar. How much the appearance of a scar bothers you is, of course, a personal matter. While no scar can be removed, we can often improve its appearance, through the injection therapy or through surgical revisions.

No scar can be removed entirely; just adjusted. The degree of improvement depends on the size and direction of your scar, the nature and quality of your skin, and how well you care for the wound after the operation

Scar Management

Keloids are thick, puckered, itchy clusters of scar tissue that grow beyond the edges of the wound or incision. They are often red or darker in color than the surrounding skin. Keloids occur when the body continues to produce the tough, fibrous protein known as collagen after a wound has healed. Keloids can appear anywhere on the body, but they are most common over the breastbone, on the earlobes, and on the shoulders. They occur more often in dark-skinned people than in those who are fair. The tendency to develop keloids lessens with age.

I treat keloids aggressively and early by injecting a steroid medication directly into the scar tissue to reduce redness, itching, and burning. In some cases, this will also shrink the scar. If steroid treatment is inadequate, the scar tissue can be cut out and the wound closed with one or more layers of stitches. This is gen-erally performed under local anesthesia as an outpatient pro-cedure. You should be back at work in a day or two, and the stitches will be removed in a few days. Unfortunately, keloids have a stubborn tendency to recur, sometimes even larger than before. I sometimes recommend the application of a pressure garment over the area for as long as a year. Keloids may return at anytime, requiring repeated procedures, but this is not common.

Hypertrophic scars are often confused with keloids, since both

Scar Reduction Methods

- Vitamin E
- Onion extract cream
- Allantoin-sulfomucopolysaccharide gel
- Glycosaminoglycan gel
- Extracts of Bulbine frutescens
- Extracts of Centella asiatica
- Topical retinoic acid
- Colchicine
- Systemic antihistamines
- Mederma

tend to be thick, red, and raised. Hypertrophic scars, however, remain within the boundaries of the original incision or wound. They often improve on their own – though it may take a year or more with the help of steroid applications or injections. If a conservative approach does not appear to be effective, hypertrophic scars can often be improved surgically. The plastic surgeon will remove excess scar tissue and may reposition the incision so that it heals in a less visible pattern. This surgery may be done under local or general anesthesia, depending on the scar's location and what you and your surgeon decide. You may receive steroid injections during surgery and at intervals for up to two years afterward to prevent the thick scar from re-forming.

Differentiating hypertrophic scars from keloids can be challenging. Scars can range between the ones that become hypertrophic in the first few months and then completely resolve with no treatment, to the keloids that become disfiguring and permanent.

Silicone gel sheeting has been a widely used option for hypertrophic scars and keloids since the 1980s. The mechanism of action of topical silicone is unknown but there are temperature differences as small as 1°C under silicone gel sheeting. This could have a profound effect on collagen kinetics and may reduce scarring. Silicone itself has never been found in significant amounts in scars treated with sheeting so a direct chemical effect is unlikely. It has also been theorized that static electricity generated by silicone gel sheeting induces a polarization of scar tissue that results in involution. Occlusion of scars by silicone gel sheeting might alter cytokine levels, which in turn would have an effect on scar remodeling.

Anne's Story

"Following my breast reduction surgery, I did have a couple of areas along my incisions that did have delayed healing. It took four to six weeks for theses areas to completely heal. As a result, I do have areas where there is thick scarring. Dr. Hurwitz introduced me to his aesthetician Molly who began laser treatments on my scars every three to six weeks. I am using a mixture of Retin A and smoothing gel and applying it to the scars. This mixture makes the top layer of skin slowly peel off, kind of like when you peel after a sun burn. I used the mixture approximately every other day depending whether I had any skin irritation from the cream. I have seen a noticeable difference in the appearance of the scars since starting this program. I have no regrets with having the surgery done and I am very pleased with the results. It has definitely had a positive impact on my life."

We have developed a graded protocol to manage postoperative scarring. I start patients using silicone gel sheeting at three to four weeks to start. The application of adhesive microporous hypoallergenic paper tape after surgery is frequently successful. The mechanism of benefit is unknown, but it may in part be mechanical (pressure therapy) and/or occlusive.

The extensive scarring that follows these procedures has been more than offset by the dramatic improvement in the body contour. While some hypertrophy, most scars fade over several years. An active scar treatment program with a variety of modalities is essential. If the scars fail to regress after eight weeks, we start a graded program with silicone sheeting, Endermologie®, microdermabrasion, topical Retin A® therapy, and intense pulsed light treatments. Adrucil (5 flurouracil) injections are occasionally used. Regardless of their appearance on the torso, the scars are usually level, symmetrical, and hidden by underwear.

Endermologie®

Endermologie® (LPG One, Inc, Miami, FL) was originally developed in France in the 1980s as a treatment for adherent scars. Adherent scars result when the skin is damaged by repeated infection or ulceration, so that scar tissue becomes attached to the skin's underlying layers. Endermologie® was developed as an alternative method to surgery for freeing the scar. In the process of freeing the scar tissue, many patients observed reduction of body dimensions and improvement in skin texture.

Since then, Endermologie® has been used as a treatment for temporary cellulite reduction and skin toning. It is a patented technique employing a mechanized device with two motorized rollers and regulated suction. This non-invasive device creates a symmetrical skin fold, which allows deep tissue mobilization to occur.

Pre-operative treatments condition soft tissues to make them more malleable and promote a more effective and efficient surgery. We have found that a course of these treatments aids in reducing recovery time and speeds swelling. After surgery, Endermologie® reduces fibrosis and scar tissue, smoothes the skin of surgical irregularities, and helps to promote healing through increased circulation, lymphatic drainage, and the elimination of fluids. We have also found that using Endermologie® in conjunction with lipoplasty may also reduce the incidence of touch-up surgeries. You will wear a body stocking as our technician gently glides the suctioning rollers over your body, concentrating on affected areas. A program of 15 to 20 35- to 45-minute relaxing sessions is recommended.

The Endermologie® system utilizes rollers and gentle suctioning to deeply massage the affected areas, increasing the circulation by 200 percent, compared with 60 percent for manual massage. Endermologie® helps your body to expel abnormal water buildup while stretching the connective fibers under the skin that have grown lax. The mechanism increases blood circulation to all parts of the body. As stiff, tense muscles are soothed, it reduces stress. Typically, the abdomen, thighs, and buttocks appear smoother and smaller after a half dozen sessions.

Manual Lymphatic Drainage (MLD)

The lymph system is the body's waste disposal system. It acts as a natural defense in the body by clearing away bacteria, cell debris, excess water, proteins, and wastes from the connective tissue back to the blood stream and ultimate removal by the kidneys. During the transportation process the lymph is cleaned, filtered, and concentrated. Many immune processes occur in the lymph nodes. If the pathways become congested, damaged, or severed, then fluids can build up in the connective tissue leading to edema, swelling, and inflammation. If there are any abnormalities in the tissues (e.g., chronic inflammation, recent surgery, congestion), it is the role of the lymphatic system to transport the damaged cells, inflammatory substances, and wasted water away from the area. The quicker this can happen, the faster recovery will be. This technique of gentle massage enhances and stimulates the lymphatic system to remove wastes more rapidly from around the cells and in the tissues, back into the lymphatic system for removal and ultimate cleansing. Dr. Emil Vodder developed MLD in France in the 1930s. He came up with a massage technique that could stimulate the pump of the lymphatic system involving gentle stationary circles on lymph nodes. MLD affects the nervous system, smoothes muscles, and increases fluid movement in the connective tissue. MLD involves a slow, rhythmical touch applied by the therapist in the form of a light massage that can be very relaxing. It has a calming, stress-reducing effect that can facilitate pain reduction.

For cellulite treatment, our medical aesthetician first assesses the condition of the skin: color, texture, temperature, moisture, and elasticity. The next step is to look at the contour of the hips and legs, and identify skin thickening, ridges, lumps, and visible scars that run across lymph vessels and may obstruct lymph drainage. She examines visible veins, looking for redness, swelling, heat, and pain. Lymphatic drainage is useful before and after body-contouring surgery to decrease bruising, edema, and inflammation.

Ultrasound Therapy

Commonly used physiotherapy externally applied ultrasound machines have been adapted for fat recontouring and post-operative care.

The therapist applies gel and places the head of the ultrasound machine on the skin. It will be gently moved in small circles. Treatment time lasts minutes. Ultrasound can be applied in two modes, continuous and pulse. Continuous ultrasound beam best transfers heat to the tissues. Pulsing reduces tissues heating.

The Cellulite Controversy

Cellulite is a disorganized pattern of skin dimpling and minor sagging of the buttocks and thighs. Sometimes likened to cottage cheese under the skin, it can be deep puckering and diffuse or like tiny pebbles under the water. Cellulite appears at any age, starting in teenagers to the onset of menopause. Often afflicting the overweight, it strikes the thin also. My patients reluctantly show me their cellulite and express despair. I am also frustrated.

It is widely accepted that some women have cellulite, and men do not. Cellulite relates to anatomy and female hormones. In women, the deep fat layer is structured as large vertical chambers, where an abundance of fat can be stored. The compartments in men are arranged as smaller diagonal units so they store less fat and are also unlikely to dimple.

Solid or firm cellulite is visible and palpable when skin is relaxed. Solid cellulite is often found on women who have probably never experienced extreme weight variations, so their tissues remain firm. Soft cellulite is not as concentrated as solid cellulite. It tends to occupy large areas, is loose, and slides easily

Cellulite Prone Areas

- Inner, outer, and posterior thighs
- Inner knees
- Upper and lower abdomen
- Hips
- Buttocks
- Lower back
- Back of upper arms
- Ankles

over muscle. Soft cellulite is only visible when the skin is pinched together between the fingers. It hangs and sags in folds and flabby bulges, and shakes like jelly with every bodily movement. When tissues lack firmness, and the skin is soft, muscle tone is poor. Soft cellulite is often found on women who have recently lost a large amount of weight. Losing weight quickly and gaining it back can exacerbate cellulite. Drastic changes in size causes tissues to lose their elasticity and firmness, becoming soft and saggy, and enabling cellulite to move to the skin's surface.

The Stages of Cellulite

Stage One The earliest formation of cellulite occurs at cellular level. Dermal deterioration is the hallmark of the first stage of cellulite formation. Blood vessel integrity breaks down, with the upper dermal region showing a loss of capillary networks. As this connective tissue deteriorates, the skin can no longer receive all of the nutrients it needs, causing even further degradation of the dermis and epidermis. Fat cells become engorged with lipid and water, often swelling to two or three times their original size.

Stage Two In the second stage, the deterioration of the tissue at the sub dermal levels is advanced. Some regions may have normal blood flow while adjacent regions can have markedly reduced blood flow. Fat cells become more engorged with lipids and clump together in the skin's fat layer. This exacerbates the blood flow problem, with the blood vessels being pushed away by the regions rich in fat deposits. Fluids tend to accumulate, increasing the variations in texture below the skin's surface. Surface lumpiness or unevenness can be visible at this stage.

Stage Three This stage is a continuation of the processes observed in Stage Two. Vascular deterioration begins to effect metabolism. Protein synthesis and repair processes are reduced which can lead to dermal thinning. Protein deposits begin to form around fatty deposits in the skin. Pinching the skin between the finger and thumb makes the "orange peel effect" easily visualized. Fibrous bands that hold them together surround fat cells. As the cells become damaged, these bands harden. With the onset of cellulite, the sub dermal fat cells become engorged with lipids and fluids and expand. The now hardened fibrous material is no longer elastic enough to expand with the fat cell. The fat begins to expand through the sides of the fibrous bands.

Stage Four This final stage of cellulite is marked by hard nodules in the dermal region, comprised of clumps of fat sur-rounded by a hard protein layer. The surface displays consid-erable irregularities, and hard nodules can be felt by pinching the skin in afflicted regions. Severe cellulite usually has been present for a number of years by the time stage four is reached. A lack of firmness is present and likely due to a deteriorated skin structure both in the epidermis and the dermal layers.

Stage Four cellulite accompanies massive weight loss. In the process of a lower body lift there is considerable improvement in the rippled skin pattern, especially in the upper thighs. Patients appreciate the return of smooth skin, which I have maximized by the addition of low term Endermologie®.

Recently highly marketed topical therapies for the treatment of sagging skin focus on the restructuring of the supporting connective tissue and vasculature through externally directed therapy. The first FDA approved treatment for the temporary correction of cellulite is Endermologie® (LPG, Miami, FL). Since the 1990s this computerized vacuum with complex motorized rollers has been manipulating fat deposits in tens of thousands of patients. There is vast clinical experience to support LPG's claim that changes in the cytoarchitecture of the subcutaneous tissue smoothes and firms thigh and buttock skin.

LPG claims that cellulite reflects:

1 Water Retention

2 Poor blood circulation

3 Fibrosis of connective tissue

4 Enlargement of fat cells

I confirm that cellulite can be improved, but the problem is inconsistency. We have been using the latest version of this machine, the Keymodule 6, for over two years and have found the suction assisted massage invaluable in accelerating post-operative recovery after body contouring surgery, including lipoplasty. Occasionally Endermologie® has assuredly reduced anticipated post-operative skin laxity after lipoplasty. At the request of the parent company, LPG has asked me to initiate clinical trials on yet a further modified machine to answer the question of indications, efficacy, and reliability of this unit for cellulite, skin laxity, and scars. In the meantime there have been modifications on this technology with the addition of near-infrared light (approximately 700 nm) and continuous-wave radio frequency.

Iontophoresis

These devices are prescription products that employ a method of using electrical currents to feed mineral salts directly into your body. They may be able to infuse an area with nutrients, but there is no proof that this works better than swallowing the same ingredient in food or in a supplement.

Dry Skin Brushing

Skin brushing is a technique in which a loofah or a body brush with natural bristles and a long handle or strap is used. Skin brushing can be carried out on wet or dry skin and should be done gently without harsh or rigorous rubbing that can damage the dermis. Its benefits are primarily exfoliation. Over-brushing will cause the skin to turn red and become irritated.

Thalassotherapy

It is well documented that sea water is rich in minerals and nutrients including iodine, copper, zinc, iron, strontium, and plankton. Thalassotherapy is a French spa technique that combines the application of seaweed and heated seawater to dilate the pores and blood vessels, making the skin more permeable and open to the absorption of sea minerals. This method has been used to treat arthritis and other medical conditions, as well as for cellulite reduction.

Lipostabil™ (Aventis)

This drug, not approved in the United States, is injected in minute amounts into the subcutaneous layer, in an attempt to reduce fat. Some physicians use Lipostabil™ alone, while others mix it with a steroid to decrease subsequent swelling. This phosphatidylcholine has been associated with nausea, diarrhea, depression, and cardiac arrhythmias.

Advocating Total Body Lift surgery for the treatment of cellulite is like killing a gnat with a sledge hammer.

Body contouring surgery improves so called soft cellulite. Let there be no misunderstanding. Advocating Total Body Lift surgery for the treatment of cellulite is like killing a gnat with a sledge hammer. There has to be an easier way. However, it is nice to know there is that added benefit.

Chapter 10

Total Body Lift™ Surgery, The Consummate Operation

Total Body Lift surgery treats sagging tissues of the torso and thighs. TBL surgery delivers optimal aesthetics following massive weight loss, aging and pregnancy. Total Body Lift surgery is more than a linked series of operations performed in one to several stages. Total Body Lift surgery is a paradigm shift from a minimal to inclusive. Total Body Lift surgery is coordinated artistic reconstruction of extensive deformity in as few stages as safely possible.

For some patients, operations of the upper and lower body are best completed in several stages. Many desire single stage Total Body Lift surgery. Appropriate candidates are young, highly motivated, and not only healthy but athletically fit. Their BMI's should be under 30. They must accept the likelihood of several unit blood transfusions. Further major procedures and some revisions are usually needed. Effectiveness and safety are intertwined and directly related to surgeon's outlook, temperament and experience. Single stage Total Body Lift surgery is bold.

Plastic surgery is all about removal of excess tissue and then creating gender specific contours. The droopiness of the mons pubis is corrected. The sensuous and sensitive mons pubis overlooks the labia majora. On profile one should see an uninterrupted gentle soft convexity from the umbilicus to the labia except for a slight rise at the coarsely haired mons pubis. Women after massive weight loss or with severe skin laxity suffer from ptosis of this neglected aspect of femininity. By removing a three sided picture frame of skin around this region and performing direct liposuction, I stretch out and sculpture the mons pubis. The new position is supported by the closure tensions from the abdominoplasty and inner thighplasty.

Similarly the progressive convexity of the feminine hips require attention to adequate fat retention despite a nearby tight suture line closure. To enlarge flattened buttocks, excess back fat can be moved to the lower buttocks. The upper arm has hanging skin and a droopy posterior fold. The oversized axillary hollow flows into lateral chest rolls. This beautiful erotic zone of complex contour changes can be reconstructed without constricting scars.

The torso is shaped by the transverse removal of excess skin, leaving level, flat, and symmetrical scars that are hidden by undergarments. The reliable positioning of the incisions that result in such favorable scars requires a consistent marking plan that includes multiple body positions, vigorous manipulation of the tissues, artistic visualization, and willingness to redraw lines until precisely right. With consistency and experience, I have gained confidence in the accuracy of the planned excisions so that there are minimal intra operative adjustments, facilitating efficiency and teamwork.

Strategic planning of the closure across the widest diameters of the torso, the inframammary folds and hips takes in some of the transverse excess. Vertical or oblique excisions of skin along the torso or thighs is reserved for special circumstances of severe gynecomastia, intervening scars, hernias, or unusually generous transverse skin and fat excess. For efficiency, an inverted midline V shaped excision is added if only a simple abdominoplasty is performed.

Since these weight loss patients suffer from inadequate skin elasticity, the closure must be as tight as possible. Over resection of skin followed by excessively tight closure of massive tissues soon leads to wound dehiscence or later to broadly depressed scars due to suture pull through, breakage, or premature disso-lution. Inadequate removal of skin and low closure tension leaves nearby feature ptosis, skin rolls, skin laxity, and/or wrinkles.

Total Body Lift surgery is analogous to craniofacial surgery. Craniofacial surgery was introduced in the 1970s as a dramatic new discipline for the congenitally deformed. I practice cranio-facial surgery. I consider it complex, high risk aesthetic facial reconstruction. Before craniofacial surgery, corrective operations for the congenitally deformed were limited in scope. Once the craniofacial approach became routine, enormous progress was made in elective facial surgery. Similarly, once I developed a routine coordinated total torso approach, the results of my body contouring improved. As I became confident in the essential elements of skin excision, I could concentrate on the aesthetic details that make a difference. Total Body Lift is as grand in scope as craniofacial surgery.

Total Body Lift surgery is a time tested way to improve the abdomen, thighs, buttocks, mid back, and breasts. Commonly, a first phase would take care of the abdomen, thighs, and lower body. I position the patient on her stomach and remove a large belt like segment of skin above the buttocks, up to the lower back. Upon closure of this gigantic wound, the thighs and buttocks are lifted. Then I turn my patient over carefully while still under anesthesia to continue with front of the thighs and abdomen. I first complete the circumferential abdominoplasty.

If it is not done immediately, I will correct the upper body deformity in Phase Two as early as three months after the first operation. My patients must wait at least three months so that most of the physical and emotional stresses of surgery are relieved. I want to be past the period of possible late infections and lower extremity thrombophlebtis. Most retained fluid should be gone. She should be ingesting a healthy diet, restoring protein stores, correcting anemia. My upper body lift consists of a reverse abdominoplasty (from umbilicus to breasts), removal of mid back rolls and reshaping of flattened and hanging breasts.

If the plan calls for single stage Total Body Lift I take out sagging skin from the mid back and upper abdomen while the patient is still prone. Most of the excess tissue can be saved as a "skinned" flap that is buried under the flattened breast for aug- mentation and shape. I take the extra time and effort to use the patient's excess skin and adipose instead of a silicone implant. The results are softer, more natural and long lasting. **(See photo gallery)**

My method hides the upper scar under the breast and along the bra line. The breasts are beautifully shaped as the nipples are raised to the optimal position. A distinct new fold is secured under the breast to help maintain breast shape and a flat upper abdomen. Often I compliment the upper body lift with my innovative L brachioplasty.

On the way to designing the Total Body Lift, I had to originate many technical details. Pre-operative marking of the intended incisions takes over 30 minutes. Instead of the traditional standing approach, I move the patient in multiple positions of lying, sitting, and standing. I use a variety of extremity positions, taking advantage of gravity to smooth out lax skin. A gender specific sculptured result is envisioned. Since I have extensive experience, I rarely change the plan during the operation, which expedites its execution. I also use only one position change to solve this circumferential deformity. This strategy helps me keep the patient's scars level and symmetrical.

I champion the technique to achieve a more effective lift of the thighs. The so-called saddlebag deformity of the outside of the thigh has been difficult to correct, especially in the massive weight loss patient. I take advantage of the law of skin laxity by utilizing a hip-hugging scar. After removing excess skin about the waist, I swing the leg out and can remove more skin than was possible in the past. When I replace the patient's leg to the operating room table, the tight skin effaces the saddlebag deformity. Precisely positioned drains under the tightly pulled outside thigh retard the formation of seromas. Deep quilting sutures also have a role. Mature seroma cavities may lead to partial recurrence of the saddlebag.

The inner thigh usually needs a lift. Often the laxity is severe enough to merit a vertical extension down the thigh. If the extra weight is not removed, the inner thigh scars may be dragged downward. I combine the inner thigh lift with the abdominoplasty and the lower body lift, despite the admonitions from luminaries in the field. The difference in my technique is that I develop superior pull throughout. (See photo gallery, pages 1, 2)

My patients are pleased to complete the entire lower body lift, abdominoplasty, and inner thigh lift in one session. I have placed scars of the L thighplasty away from view in a bathing suit as much as possible.

I have designed an upper body lift that improves the mid torso, upper abdominal skin rolls, and pancakes breasts, leaving behind scars hidden under a brassiere. Excess skin is turned into flaps of tissue to enlarge and reshape the breasts. I complete the upper body transformation with my L brachioplasty. I remove excess skin and fat of the upper arm, axilla, and side of the chest roughly in the form of an L. The scar may take many months to mature, leaving a sweeping and as inconspicuous scar as possible.

For severe male gynecomastia, I pioneered the boomerang excision of two narrow ellipses, draped around the nipple areolar complex. The outer ellipse continues through removal of the back roll. Those chest scars take over a year to fade. It is better if the chest is hairy to obscure what scar remains. (See photo gallery, page 21)

As soon as the Upper Body Lift was developed, measures were instituted to improve its safety. By implementing a consistent and logical plan, we have been able to gain efficiency and improve the surgical outcomes. Attentive in-hospital three days of post-operative care allows for the early discovery of healing and medical problems so they can be treated. The support of Magee Women's Hospital of the University of Pittsburgh Medical Center has been instrumental in keeping our complications low.

My patients want optimal cosmetic results in as few stages as possible with acceptable risk. I have found many ways to increase efficiency and improve safety in these long operations. It starts with devotion and attention to a busy body contouring practice. Next, I organized a dedicated team. On every case, two experienced operators assist me as I move from one area to another removing more excess skin.

Efficiencies are gained by a consistent and logical plan with only one patient turn. Accurate fluid management, and conservative blood replacement, anti-embolism prophylaxis and patient warming are essential. The latest equipment and technology is readily available. My operations are a study in time usage and efficiency. Like the concert pianist that conducts the orchestra, I must perform and lead the team through complex surgery. Reducing a nine hour operation to seven hours is accomplished through team work and reduces patient trauma as well as hastening recovery. Finally, I inject solutions containing vasoconstrictors and local anesthetic, which decreases bleeding, and reduces the need for tissue damaging electrocautery. The local anesthetic reduces early post-operative pain. Immediately your intravenous line will be connected to a narcotic pain control infusion under your control. Intravenous antibiotics may be continued for several days.

Recovery Time

It takes about four weeks to recover from Total Body Lift surgery. Early recovery is in a tertiary care hospital. After several hours in an advanced recovery room the patient is transferred to a beautifully furnished well-staffed private hospital room in a post-surgical unit. High quality residents as well as skilled and understanding nursing care are available around the clock. If a patient's condition deteriorates, transfer to an Intensive Care Unit is immediate for continuous monitoring and care. Usually the stay is three days. Intermittent pressure stockings help prevent dreaded thrombophlebitis and allow for comfortable bed rest for the first 16 hours. Continuous monitoring of fluid intake and output through an indwelling bladder catheter and suction drains are essential.

Some excess water retention due to traumatic swelling and stress hormone release is expected over several weeks. When the patient's condition is stable and can freely walk around on her own, the bladder catheter is removed. Prior to discharge the patient will be washed and sent home in properly sized elastic garments.

After discharge, we encourage our patients to increase progressively non-taxing light activity. Within four weeks most patients can resume daily functions, such as driving and deskwork. Elastic garments are worn for six weeks to encourage proper healing and provide support for the incisions. The first office visit is ten days after surgery. The dramatic improvement in body contour is evident. Stitches around the umbilicus are removed. I will remove suction drains with low out put. Many patients can resume vigorous exercise after six weeks.

Who Can Benefit from Total Body Lift Surgery?

1 The first group has excess skin in the belly, hips, thighs, and sagging buttocks. These changes are common in the mid-30 to 50-something group. They are associated with reduced skin laxity due to aging, and secondary to changes from multiple pregnancies. Baby boomers are not as tolerant of figure faults as prior generations. Reality television has increased the acceptance of life altering surgery.

2 The second group carries extra weight around the trunk. Many have attempted for years to lose their excess poundage but are unable to. A traditional abdominoplasty may be inadequate, especially in the hip, flank, and buttocks areas. Their fat distribution requires extensive liposuction prior to or during body-contouring surgery. Ultrasonic assisted lipoplasty, (I prefer the Vaser™ system of LipoSelection℠) plays a major role in the least traumatic method fat removal.

3 The third group has had massive weight loss following intestinal bypass surgery or drastic life style improvement. Most have lost more than 100 pounds. They typically will have hanging skin and fat in the area of the abdomen, outer thigh excess, hip excess that may hang, back rolls, and ill-defined buttocks. Many of these patients are disheartened when they

come to see the plastic surgeon. They have worked hard to lose all of the weight, but still cannot wear normal clothing in the hanging skin deprive them of a normal contour.

According to the American Society of Aesthetic Plastic Surgery, "the number of body lifts will increase, as post-bariatric surgery patients seek plastic surgery to rid themselves of the excess skin left hanging after massive weight loss." This correlates with the findings from the American Society of Bariatric Surgery, which indicates "that gastric bypass surgery jumped last year to more than 103,000," leading to a significant increase in demand for body contouring procedures.

Some individuals are not good candidates for Total Body Lift surgery. The morbidly obese (BMI over 40 or 35 with significant co-morbidities) are not accepted. Contour improvement will be modest, and the healing can be problematic. Patients with chronic unresolved medical problems that place them in Class III ASA risk need medical tuning prior to this major surgery. In addition, patients who are deemed mentally unable to handle an extensive surgical procedure and recovery are not appropriate. If they respond to counseling and psychotropic medications, then they may be reconsidered.

For some patients, correcting poor nutritional status is critical. Tip offs are recurrent vomiting, food intolerances, and lower extremity edema. My experienced staff nutritionist covers the issues of malnutrition and initiates therapy. The procedure may be delayed for patients planning to lose more weight.

Unlike my patients in the 1980s, baby boomers today do not accept the pancake breast deformity. They also want their breast and upper body deformity corrected together. In fact with the techniques just described, the patients' breasts for the first time become attractive. They will have naturally shaped soft, stable, and full sized breasts that merge into the reshaped axilla that balance the lower body. This unforeseen breast improvement helps compensate for the enormous effort and aesthetic short-comings. They are amazed that their own flabby tissue can be recycled to create beautiful breasts.

The extensive scarring that follows these procedures has been more than offset by the dramatic improvement in the breasts, torso, and arms. While some patients have scars that become raised or irregular, most will fade over several years. An active scar treatment program with a variety of modalities is essential.

"People now find that I am funny and fun to be around. I was before but they just didn't bother to find out. They say I am beautiful. I was before but they just didn't look. They say I am happier now. I was happy before, but it's just so hard to show happiness when people you deal with don't see or hear you. I always got the feeling from people that I was not worth listening to. People speak to me now who never did before. People are friendlier and nicer. Now I can sit anywhere and I fit into any clothes I like. Yes, I am happier now, because the world around me wants to know me for who I am. I am worth listening to. It makes life so much easier and healthier." – Sue

Itemizing the Costs

Total Body Lift surgery is complex, high risk, and life affirming. Understandably, there are considerable direct and indirect costs. First, there is the surgeon's fee. Then there are the separate hospital and anesthesia charges. There are also travel and lodging costs in Pittsburgh. Time away from work should also be factored.

Magee Women's Hospital offers discounted charges for the operating room, anesthesia services and hospital stay. The fees

Body Contouring Surgical Fees*

Procedure	Surgical Fee Range
Upper body lift	$8,000 to $12,000
Circumferential abdominoplasty	$6,000 to $12,000
Lower body lift	$10,000 to $14,000
Upper inner thighplasty	$3,500 to $6,000
L (vertical extended) inner thighplasty	$5,000 to $12,000
Pubic monsplasty	$2,000 to $6,000
Spiral flap breast augmentation/shaping	$6,000 to $10,000
Breast augmentation with implants	$3,500 to $$5,000
Breast lift or reduction	$2,000 to $5,000
Armlift (L brachioplasty)	$4,000 to $8,000
Lipoplasty and UAL	$3,000 per area
Single stage Total Body Lift surgery	$30,000 to $60,000
Facelift, eyelidplasty and browlift	$15,000 to $25,000

An itemized statement is prepared at the first office visit. Combining component operations may reduce the charge per procedure. For instance, a breast lift with implant augmentation may cost approximately $6,000 instead of $7,000. An estimate can also be conveyed over the Internet (www.hurwitzcenter.com) or by telephone.

are based on the number of hours, the complexity, and the number of the procedures. In 2004, the operating room costs in Pittsburgh were approximately $500 per hour. Anesthesia fees are determined in a similar fashion. For example, the charges for ten hours in the operating room and three days in the hospital might average a total of about $5,000.

We have no fixed schedule of operative fees. Since there is considerable variation in the presentation of patients and the component operations of Total Body Lift surgery, it is impossible to be precise. The surgical fee reflects experience, innovation, artistry, and skill. It also includes the services of my staff in the office and the operating room. Larger patients, over 200 pounds, will take longer; smaller patients often have higher expectations.

Total Body Lift surgery usually consists of an abdominoplasty, lower body lift, bilateral medial thighplasties (or vertical thighplasty), and upper body lift with breast reshaping. This surgery is performed in one, two, or three stages. Bilateral arm lift is an added procedure. Some patients have a facelift, eyelids, and browlift.

Fees for lipoplasty are based on the amount to be removed, the number of areas to be sculpted, and the goals of the patient. The charges tend to be reduced when there are coincidental procedures, such as a breast lift or a facelift.

I do not base my choice of staging on financial considerations. However, there is immense value to the patient of a one-stage operation. Theoretically the risk is greater, but I did not see that upon retrospective study of my cases, although single stage patients did receive more blood transfusions.

If the reader wishes to learn the average fees for each of these procedures charged across the United States, I refer them to the statistics posted on www.surgery.org, the official website of the American Society for Aesthetic Plastic Surgery. I caution that those fees do not reflect the charges of the most prominent surgeons in major markets.

Some candidates that see me for Total Body Lift surgery are astounded by the costs. They may be higher than anything they have ever purchased, except perhaps a car or a home. It takes intense reflection on priorities and values to commit such personal resources or indebtedness. For some, transformational surgery is the most important event in their lives and the gateway to improved esteem, social, and financial success. It validates the decision for bariatric surgery in the first place. For loved ones there is no limit to affording a safe recovery. Sometimes operative staging is necessary for purely financial limitations.

"Sometimes I go by a mirror and I have to stare because I still don't believe it is me. My inner person still has not changed. I am the Deirdre that I used to be 20 years ago, and she is something! I am not a pushover anymore. I'm not hiding behind my weight. And I'm not at the sidelines!" – Deirdre

Informed Consent–Weighing the Risks

Informed consent for surgery follows a process of physician and staff education with interaction. This book gives extensive, but generalized information. Informed consent may be given by the patient after a personalized treatment plan is proposed. That individualized plan is possible only after an appropriate history, physical examination, testing, and assessment.

At the initial consultation I will introduce the concepts, components, and risks of Total Body Lift surgery. We have a chance to discuss all the issues in great detail. Reading this book should prepare you well, although I have formulated a personalized eight page office informed consent document that summarizes what the patient needs to know.

Plastic surgery is a service not a product. The results cannot be guaranteed. Even experience and attention to organization and technical detail do not ensure a result that can only be imagined by me and the patient. Our patient coordinator will show prospective patients many before and after photographs to inform

them of the improvements, scars, and limitations, of these procedures. They are also routinely invited to talk to prior patients to
learn of their experiences and personal insights. They are also
given a detailed educational video presentation.

Reversionary procedures are indicated when the final result
falls short of expectations. There could have been an error in
technique or problematic healing. There must be agreement
between the patient and the surgeon that the revision is appropriate. Revision surgery is common in cosmetic surgery. In the
centerfold there is an example of the addition of scar revision and
further liposuction that made a substantial improvement of a very
good result. **(See photo gallery, page 31)**

---

*"I was fast approaching 300 pounds when I made the decision to
take back charge of my life and I was successful. Inches and pounds
were gone but I still felt like a prisoner in my sagging, hanging body.
I heard about the work that Dr. Hurwitz was doing, did my
homework, and scheduled a consultation. I knew the day I first met
him that I was in the right place. Dr. Hurwitz told me "I like what I
do and I'm very good at it" and he backed up what he told me with
pictures. I was treated with the utmost respect as he examined,
tugged, pulled, and photographed me…naked! Never once was I
embarrassed or feel like I was on display.*

*In November 2003 I had my upper body restored to normalcy
followed just four short months later by my lower body. My results
are fantastic, and I like the way I look. People ask, would you do it
again? You bet! As a matter of fact in December 2004 I returned
for a third procedure to lean out my middle section. It was about
comfort, I couldn't keep my pantyhose up!*

*I am now one month out from that surgery and it's all good.
Not only do my pantyhose stay up but I look great! An entire
lifetime of my "midriff bulge" issue is gone. Three major surgeries
in 13 months meant a huge commitment and took a lot of perse-*

verance but that's what I needed to do after massive weight loss. I set a goal over two years ago, kept my focus on the end result and I'm there. I will always be so very grateful for the part that the good Dr. Hurwitz did to help me get to where I am today. I am healthy, I feel great and I look fantastic!" – Cathy

Risks

Every operation entails the risk of problems or unwanted events. The choice to have a procedure should be based on the comparison of likely benefit to probable risk.

Change in Plans Since Total Body Lift surgery is complex, there may necessary major changes in plans during the operation, which may be unforeseen. Giving consent to a procedure does not mean that it will be performed exactly as anticipated.

Bleeding Due to the extensive nature of these operations, you are likely to lose enough blood to warrant transfusions. In Pittsburgh that means volunteer donated blood from the hospital blood bank. Depending on your blood count, you may donate up to two units of blood in the month prior to surgery. Rarely there is excessive bleeding during or after the operation. Should postoperative bleeding occur, you may require emergency treatment to drain accumulated blood and further blood transfusions. If you absolutely wish to minimize the chance for a transfusion, then choose multiple operative sessions.

Infection Infections range from troublesome to dangerous. Minor wound infections, accompanied by exposed and "spitting" sutures are common and are usually treated by limited debridement and dressing care. Minor infection may spread to cellulitis or abscess.

Major infection has fever and you feel sick like the flu. Such signs and symptoms require an investigation. Should you have an infection, you are prescribed intravenous antibiotics and perhaps additional surgery to remove dead tissue and drain pus. Theoretically, there is a greater risk of infection when multiple body-contouring procedures are combined in one stage

Change in Nipple and Skin Sensation You may experience a change in the sensitivity of the nipples and the skin of your breasts. Permanent loss of nipple sensation, excessive sensitivity, or pain can occur in one or both nipples.

Long Term Effects Subsequent alterations in body contour may occur as the result of aging, weight loss or gain, pregnancy, or other circumstances unrelated to the above procedures.

Pain Chronic pain may occur, probably from nerves becoming trapped in scar tissue.

Sutures Sutures may spontaneously poke through the skin, be visible, or produce irritation that requires removal. Since sutures are used to tighten abdominal muscle fascia and narrow the abdomen, their ability to hold the abdomen flat are not assured. Therefore unwanted post-operative abdominal fullness may occur.

Anesthesia Both local and general anesthesia involve risks, which will be discussed by your anesthesiologist on the day of surgery. Regardless of your health, there are complications, injury, and death from anesthesia.

  Local Local anesthetic agents temporarily block nerves from carrying pain signals to the brain. The injection may be given directly into the area to be operated on or around the main trunks of regional sensory nerves. Another form of local anesthetic is a topical or surface form such as a spray, gel, or cream

applied to the area to be numbed. Some of these forms have to
be left on the skin to penetrate for 30 minutes or longer before
treatment. There is no loss of consciousness with local anesthesia,
so patients are able to communicate with the physician and an
anesthesiologist is not present.

Regional Regional anesthesia involves the injection of a local
anesthetic to provide numbness, loss of pain, or loss of sensation
to a large region of the body. Regional anesthetic techniques
include spinal blocks and epidural blocks which are usually supplemented with sedatives relieve anxiety and cause drowsiness.

Twilight (Monitored Anesthesia Care) Cosmetic procedures are
often performed under local anesthesia with the addition of
'twilight' or a sedative given intravenously, such as Valium or
Versed, so you can be thoroughly relaxed. These medications
supplement local anesthetic injections, which are usually given by
your cosmetic surgeon. You will be in a sleepy state, but may
drift in and out of consciousness. This allows the direct area
being operated on to be numbed, while you are relaxed, but not
as heavily sedated as you would be with a general anesthesia. An
anesthesia provider provides the sedation and monitors all bodily
functions as if you were receiving a general anesthetic.

General A general anesthetic provides loss of consciousness
and loss of sensation, and is commonly used in larger surgical
procedures where the body may sustain a substantial amount of
trauma, or if multiple procedures are being performed. A general
anesthetic is administered by injection, gas, or a combination of
both and causes you to fall into a deep sleep. A breathing tube is
inserted to protect your airway and provide the inhalation agents.
This tube is removed at the end of the procedure. Other drugs
are used to take away all sensations and relax your muscles. The
anesthesia provider puts you to sleep by giving you a small
injection of rapidly acting drugs.

Only board certified anesthesiologists who teach at the
University of Pittsburgh Medical Center are entrusted to care for

my patients. Anesthesia affects your entire system. It is important that you inform your anesthesiologist of your medical condition, medications, herbal supplements, and any previous adverse anesthesia experiences.

Our medical staff will take a complete medical history prior to surgery. The final clearance before surgery actually rests in the hands of the anesthesiologist who will review your records to ensure that you are fit for surgery and anesthesia. If your blood pressure is elevated, if you have a chest infection, if you are running a fever, or if you have reversible laboratory abnormalities, your surgery will be postponed until these problems are corrected. Your anesthesiologist manages your medical situation arising during surgery, watching for flare ups of chronic medical conditions such as asthma, diabetes, high blood pressure, or heart failure.

Allergic Reactions In rare cases, local allergies to tape, suture material, or topical preparations have been reported. Systemic reactions which are more serious may occur with drugs used during surgery and prescription medications.

Aesthetic Shortcomings Surgery is an imperfect science, and you may be disappointed with the results. Under treatment leaves residual laxity and looseness. Over treatment leaves excessive tightness of skin, with flattening of regional contours and widening of scars. Some loose tissue remains because the torso skin laxity also occurs in the horizontal direction, which is not fully treated. Considerable judgment is used to achieve the optimum shape and skin turgor, but for a variety of reasons the ultimate aesthetics may be suboptimal and that risk must also be understood. Excessive firmness of the breast can occur after surgery due to internal scarring or scarring around a breast implant if one is used. The ultimate symmetry, size, and shape of your reconstructed breasts are unpredictable due to the complexity of the operation.

Pregnancy/Breast Feeding Concerns Mastopexy, breast reshaping, and reduction may interfere with breast feeding. Following pregnancy, your breast skin may stretch and offset the results of the breast reshaping.

Making the Right Choice for You

Once all the indicated surgical procedures are identified, the expenses, time commitments, and risks are reviewed. Then a surgical plan is coordinated so that as many procedures as possible can be done simultaneously. If you qualify for a single stage TBL there are great advantages over multiple stages, but theoretically you are assuming increased risk. My surgeon detractors admonish that ten hour elective reconstructive operations are an expression of exuberance, perhaps testosterone excess. That if I were putting patient safety first I would divide up the operation into multiple stages. They say, "What's the rush?" They say cosmetic operations should not take so long. In response, I reject my choice of a single stage body lift as macho behavior. Nevertheless, I do admit exhilaration when finishing these complex efforts and seeing a beautiful body take form. My quality results and safety are a matter of record. My highly skilled anesthesiologists are understanding and fully cooperative. No one is disturbed as colleagues at my University take just as long to reconstruct craniofacial malformation in children or replace a cancerous breast with a microvascular transfer of a free flap. Some patients give you one good shot. They will not return to the operating room for another major procedure. I have found a synergism in these procedures. Minor wound healing problems are common regardless of the number of stages. I remain a vigilant observer and will continue to offer single stage reconstruction to good candidates who value a single stage until results prove otherwise.

I think it is most appropriate to end this experiential book with the words from one of my own patients, Jennifer, whose story can be found in Chapter Two. **(See photo gallery, page 6)**

"As I lay in my hospital bed on the night of my third, and probably last, operation, I had an amazing feeling of freedom wash over me. 'Freedom' was not an emotion I had expected to feel. But, indeed, I did feel free – I was finally free of all the restrictions my body had placed on my soul. I was free to move on, to go wherever I wanted to go, to do whatever I wanted to do. For the first time ever, I was free. A lifetime of wanting things that I dared not even hope for was over. The tears I shed then were not for the physical pain I was experiencing – they were tears of happiness. I don't think I had realized before the extent to which my body had held me back. No more. I really felt like a new person. What a long, sometimes frightening, and yet an amazing journey I had been on. Had I known what was ahead, would I have had gastric bypass surgery in the beginning? I surely hope so. Had I not started the journey, I would have never, in my whole life, achieved freedom.

"The person, who led me on this journey to freedom, was Dr. Hurwitz. He made me feel like I was worth the effort on his part (my severe skin issues were a great challenge to him), and that what had been impossible all my life was now possible. In a very realistic way, he encouraged me. He helped me get over the feeling that cosmetic surgery is a vain thing; that it is done by people who think solely about themselves. He also didn't give up on me when things didn't go well – my legs required surgery three times and he undertook each surgery with hope that they would improve. He did not charge me for the second and third attempts; he said the success of my leg operations were as important to him as they were to me. His care was exceptional. His doctoring benefited me physically, but he also healed my spirit and led me emotionally. I will be forever grateful to him, and I will never forget him or his abilities. He is a fine, fine surgeon, a gifted artist, and a lovely human being."

Glossary

A

Abduction: Outward or away from the body positioning of an extremity

Abdominoplasty: Commonly known as a tummy tuck, is a major surgical procedure to remove excess skin and fat from the middle and lower abdomen and to tighten the muscles of the abdominal wall.

Abscess: A localized collection of pus usually infected and caused by bacteria.

Adipose tissue: A complex layer of fat cells, connective tissue, and neurovasculature.

Adjustable gastric banding: Also known as the lap band, a small, silicone ring is placed around the stomach near the esophagus to limit food intake, using a laparoscopic approach. It has a thin silicone tube extension that connects to a fill dome placed just under the abdominal skin. Sterile water is injected into the dome to increase or decrease the constriction caused by the ring.

Anti-inflammatory: A substance known to counteract inflammation or swelling.

Areola: The naturally dark round pigmented area that surrounds the projecting nipple.

Arnica Montana: A botanical derived from a mountain plant with antiseptic, astringent, antimicrobial and anti-inflammatory properties.

Autogenous: Reconstructive material originating from one's own tissues

Axillae: (plural of axilla) The armpit or the cavity beneath the junction of the arm and shoulder.

B

Bicep: The large flexor muscle of the front of the upper arm and back of the upper leg.

Biliopancreatic diversion: A composite repositioning of the upper intestines.

Body Mass Index (BMI): A measure of body fat that is the ratio of the weight of the body in kilograms to the square of its height in meters. A body mass index that exceeds a value of 25 indicates overweight. BMI between 30 and 35 is considered obese; over 35 is severely obese; and over 40 is morbidly obese.

Arm lift: Also known as a brachioplasty, this operation reduces the skin redundancy and fat volume; thereby improving the contour and shape of the upper arm leaving as few and inconspicuous scars as possible. It has a variably long scar along the inner aspect of the arm

Bromelain: A protease obtained from the juice of the pineapple.

Buccal fat pad: A pad of cheek fat lying lateral to the lips and below the cheek bone. It remains rather large and descends into the jowls after weight loss and aging.

Buttock Crease: Lower fold of the buttocks.

C

Cannulae: Long, thin hollow tubular instrument with side openings near one end and a connection to high pressure suction machine on the other which is used to extract fat by vigorous back and forth motion during liposuction

Cellulite: A dimpled and irregular contour pattern of skin variably present in the buttocks and thighs of aging women, thought to be due to deposits of fat, toxins, and fluids trapped in pockets beneath the skin.

Cellulitis: Diffuse bacterial infection of the fatty layer under the skin. When the bacteria are virulent, the infection can rapidly spread and lead to gangrene, which is tissue death.

Circumferential: Completely around a surface, as in a belt excision around the lower abdomen.

Colle's Fascia: The strong deep subcutaneous fascia or layer deep to the external labia or scrotum.

D

Debridement: The surgical removal of devitalized and/or infected tissue due to injury or disease. Limited debridement can be performed in the office as cutting stops at bleeding or sensate tissue.

Deep vein thrombosis: The presence of a blood clot within a deeply positioned vein of the lower trunk or legs. This is the source of life threatening pulmonary embolism or clots that may flow upward to the lung veins after major operations.

Dehiscence: The separation of the sutured edges of a surgical wound. It can be superficial (skin deep) or complete (down to muscular fascia).

Dermis: The thicker layer of skin under the superficial epithelial cover called the epidermis. It imparts to skin strength through collagen and elasticity through elastin. The hair follicles, sweat glands, blood vessels and nerves reside in this deeper layer of skin.

Diabetes: An altered state of sugar metabolism due to insensitivity to (type 2) or lack of insulin hormone (type 1). Type 2 is common in obesity and leads to a variety of disorders of the cardiovascular system, nervous system and skin, now called the metabolic syndrome.

Digestion: The process of making food absorbable by dissolving it and breaking it down into simpler chemical compounds that occurs in the living body chiefly through the action of enzymes secreted into the alimentary canal.

Drain: A plastic multiperforated tube, connected to a compressible vacuum bulb, which is placed under skin flaps for a week or two to collect blood and serum. Premature remoVaser Assisted Lipoplasty may lead to a seroma.

Duodenum: The first, shortest, and widest part of the small intestine that in humans is about 10 inches (25 centimeters) long and that extends from the pylorus to the undersurface of the liver where it descends for a variable distance and receives the bile and pancreatic ducts and then bends to the left and finally upward to join the jejunum near the second lumbar vertebra.

E

Edema: An abnormal excess accumulation of serous fluid in connective tissue, such as ankle swelling or in a serous cavity, such as pulmonary congestion.

Endermologie®: A proprietary method made by LPG of reducing post-operative edema, and temporarily smoothing cellulite and loose skin by a high tech roller massage and vacuum system.

Epidermis: The superficial protective layer of skin containing a maturing layer of epithelial cells including melanocytes, which impart color. It overlies the dermis.

Epigastrium: The part of the abdominal wall above the umbilicus (belly button). The hypogastrium is the part of the abdominal wall below the umbilicus. The abdominal wall can be divided into upper and lower halves; or it can be further divided into quadrants by drawing a vertical line through the umbilicus.

Extrusion: The erosion of skin that allows an implant (chin, lip, breast, etc.) to become exposed. Once an implant becomes exposed, it should be removed before the inevitable extrusion.

F

Fascia: The sheet of firm connective tissue that covers muscles, sometimes used as a graft material.

Fat Embolus: Particles of fat that access the bloodstream during surgery and then spread to the lungs and when enough emboli are released there will be shortness of breath and chest pain. The emboli may pass through the lungs to have adverse effects on brain or kidney function even leading to death.

Flap of skin: A composite segment of continuously vascularized skin and fat that is moved from its natural location to another through incision release of restricting tissue.

G

Gallstones: A calculus (stone) formed in the gallower body liftadder or biliary passages.

General Anesthesia: Commonly referred to as being asleep. A total loss of consciousness induced through inhalation of special gases by an anesthetist (nurse) or anesthesiologist (physician). Your breathing is usually controlled through a tube placed in your airway and you won't feel anything. Supplemental intravenous narcotics and local anesthesia reduce surgical site pain upon awakening.

Gynecomastia: Development of female like breasts on a male. Its treatment is complicated by sagging inelastic skin. Liposuction and chest wall skin excision are the common treatments.

H

HCG: Human chorionic gonadotropin, a human hormone made by chorionic cells in the fetal part of the placenta. The presence of HCG is detectable by immunologic means within days of fertilization and forms the foundation of the common pregnancy tests. The level of HCG tends to be higher with a female fetus soon after conception.

Hematoma: A mass of clotted blood that forms in a tissue, organ, or body space as a result persistent bleeding from injured blood vessels. Enlarging hematomas may be painful and must be evacuated by opening nearby incisions and removing the excess fluid. Smaller hematomas are allowed to liquefy and are aspirated a week or so later.

Hernia: A protrusion of an organ or part through connective tissue or through a wall of the cavity in which it is normally enclosed. Because of the excessive weight in patients with large incision bariatric surgery, there is a greater than 50% rate of incisional hernias of the abdominal wall.

Hyperpigmentation: Darkening of the skin through overproduction of melanin by melanocytes. Post solar irradiation hyperpigmentation is the common sun tan. Tanning recent surgical scars often leads to unwanted permanent darkening.

Hypertension: Abnormally high arterial blood pressure, common in obesity and leads to severe cardiovascular occlusive disease, kidney insufficiency, stroke and premature death.

Hyperplasia: Enlarged volume through increase in umber of cells. In children fat stores can enlarge by multiplying adipocytes.

Hypertrophic scar: A thickened, elevated and red scar that fails to reduce in size over several months.

Hypertrophy: Enlarged volume through gain in cellular size. In adults fat stores usually enlarge by each adipose cell gaining fat.

I

Informed Consent: A process of educating a patient with a reasonable amount of information regarding their treatment, alternatives to that treatment and risks of adverse events and complications.

Inframammary fold: The skin fold that lies at the base of the breast and above the abdomen. Sagging breasts drape over this fold. Your brassiere should fit snuggly against it.

Intertrigo: The inflammatory skin condition due to maceration and infection under moisten folds of skin, commonly experienced after massive weight loss.

J

Jejunum: The first half of the small intestine

Jowls: Bulging laxity along the jaw lines lateral to the chin

K

Keloid: Enlarged, permanent and thickened skin scar that extends beyond the original injury in a mushroom manner. It is more common in dark skin, and often familial.

L

Lap Band Adjustable Gastric Banding: An inflatable plastic restrictive ring placed around the proximal stomach that variably restricts good intake.

Laparoscope: A rigid tubular structure that contains lenses and fiber optic cable that emits high intensity light and transmits video images of intra abdominal anatomy. It is placed through a stab wound through the abdominal wall.

Laparoscopic Surgery: Operations performed within the abdominal cavity through multiple portals and gas insufflations by means of a laparoscope and specially designed instruments.

Lateral Thigh: Part of the thigh situated on the outer side

Laxity: The quality or state of being loose

M

Malabsorption: Faulty absorption of nutrient materials from the alimentary canal

Mastopexy: Breast lift procedure that improves the shape of the breast with nipple elevation.

Medial Thigh: The inner portion of the thighs

Minimally Invasive Surgery: Operations performed through smaller incisions than in the past through the use of endoscopes, high quality magnified video and remote instrumentation.

Mons Pubis: A hairy, rounded eminence upon the pubic area

N

Necrosis: Tissue death usually due to inadequate blood supply.

Nipple Areola Complex: The nipple and the surrounding areola.

O

Obesity: A condition characterized by excessive body fat and directly related chronic metabolic disorders such as diabetes. The most accepted measure of obesity is BMI over 30.

Off label use: The prescribed use of a drug or medical devise by a medical practitioner for an indication not approved by the Federal Drug Administration.

P

Panniculectomy: Surgical excision of redundant pannus or section of skin and fat of the abdomen.

Parasternal: Near the junction of the sternum (breast plate) and the ribs.

Pectoralis Major Muscle: A large flat muscle immediately under the breast that extends from the first seven ribs to the upper arm humerus bone.

Periareolar: Refers to a concentric excision circle around the areola used for mastopexy.

Peritoneum: The smooth transparent serous membrane that lines the cavity of the abdomen, is folded inward over the abdominal and pelvic viscera, and consists of an outer layer closely adherent to the walls of the abdomen and an inner layer that folds to invest the viscera.

Peritonitis: Infection of the peritoneum usually due to injury of the intestines with leakage of contents.

Plication: Overlapping tissue through the proper placement and tying of sutures.

Prone: Lying face down on one's stomach

Ptosis: Relating to or affected with the sagging of a structure or an organ

Pulmonary Embolus: A blockage of an artery in the lungs by fat, air, tumor tissue, or blood clot

R

Reduction Mammoplasty: The removal of excess breast tissue, followed by repositioning of the nipple and flap reconstruction to improve the shape.

Reverse Abdominoplasty: Removing excess skin and improving upper abdominal contour through an incision along the inframammary folds and creation of an undermined inferiorly based abdominal skin pedicle.

Roux-en-Y gastric bypass: A technique of intestinal realignment that leaves a small stomach pouch attached to a limb of small intestine that bypasses the remaining stomach, duodenum, proximal jejunum. The altered intestinal alignment forms a Y.

S

Saddlebags: The bulging and sagging skin along the upper outer thighs in women

Septae: A dividing wall or membrane between bodily spaces or masses of soft tissue

Seroma: A pool of clear fluid called serum lying under the skin most often following operations that leave large spaces such as flap and liposuction surgery. The prolonged use of surgical drains reduces the incidence of this complication. It is treated by aspiration.

Silicone: A chemical polymer of alternating silicon and oxygen atoms processed to a gel form to fill silicone elastomer breast implants. Also it is used off label in a liquid injectable form for facial contour depressions.

Silicone elastomer: Synthetic heat cured silicone that may be solid for chin, cheek, pectoral or calf implants or formed into an inflatable bag, which is placed under the breasts and then filled to the desired volume with saline.

Sleep apnea: Intermittent periods of brief cessation of breathing during sleep. It is caused in the obese by obstruction of the airway and is associated with excessive daytime sleepiness and irritability. When chronic and severe it leads to pulmonary hypertension, congestive heart failure, and even death.

SMAS: an acronym for Superficial Musculo Aponeurotic System. It is a firm layer of tissue that covers the superficial muscles in the cheek and extends over the lower face and neck muscle called the platysma.

SFS: an acronym for Superficial Fascial System. It is a multilayered organized collagenous layer of the subcutaneous tissue that is carefully preserved and sutured together under tension during body-contouring surgery.

Sternal Notch: It lies at the top of the sternum at the midline base of the neck

Striae: Commonly known as stretch marks, they are parallel striae of dermal thinning usually in areas of rapid enlargement during hormone changes, such as the lower abdomen during pregnancy. They initially appear as a series red, raised lines, and then turn purple. Over years they widen and depress to form reflective whitened striae.

Subcutaneous Tissue: The variably thick composite connective and adipose tissue between the skin and muscular fascia. The adipose imparts skins softness, pliability, surface contour and body warmth and protection.

Supine: Lying face up, flat on one's back

Suture: A strand or fiber used to sew together parts of the living body. Permanent sutures do not dissolve and absorbable sutures do disappear in time.

T

Thighplasty: An operation to reduce the skin redundancy and adipose volume; and thereby, improve the contour and shape of the thigh leaving as few and inconspicuous scars are possible. The lower body lift improves the outer thigh and a medial thighplasty raises the inner thigh.

Tumescent Infiltration: A method to provide tissue numbness and decrease bleeding prior to incisions and liposuction. Small amounts of xylocaine for local anesthesia and epinephrine for vasoconstriction are added to large volumes of saline which is then infiltrated into the operative regions until the tissues are sufficiently swollen.

Turgor: The fullness or tension produced by the fluid content of blood vessels, capillaries, and cells.

U

Ultrasonic Assisted Lipoplasty: The use of ultrasound technology to emulsify subcutaneous fat, followed by traditional liposuction.

Ultrasound: Application under the skin of a rapidly oscillating probe that emits sound like a tuning fork at a wave frequency of 27 kilohertz, which is too high to be audible. Fat cells are selectively vulnerable to the disruptive effects of this mechanical vibration.

Umbilicus: Belly button or navel

Umbilicoplasty: Operative creation of a new or modified umbilicus

V

Vaser: A second generation ultrasound device delivering energy with a patented pulsed waveform and uniquely designed probe emulsifies adipose tissue as effectively as alternative instruments but with a reduction in power. Less power results in less thermal injury to remaining tissues.

Vertical banded gastroplasty: A food restrictive operation through significantly narrowing of the stomach by partitioning a side unusable pouch.

Vertical Pattern Breast Lift: A method of breast lifting involving the removal of skin in a vertical direction followed by medial and lateral breast tissue approximation.

W

Wise Pattern Mastopexy: Brassiere like pattern for breast reduction introduced by Houston Plastic Surgeon Robert Wise in 1957. Also referred to as an anchor pattern mastopexy, a key hole pattern is centered over the nipple areolar complex with the top of the pattern being the location of the new position. The lower ends of the key hole extended outward to the inner and outer aspects of the breast and are met by an incision along the inframammary fold. The final scar is in the shape of an anchor.

X

Xyphoid: The lower most portion of the sternum, which is the upper most extent of Abdominoplasty dissection

Z

Z-Plasty: The transposition of adjoining triangular flaps in the form of the letter Z

Resources

- www.hurwitzcenter.com
- www.usalipo.com
- www.totalbodyliftsurgery.com
- www.plasticsurgery.org
- www.surgery.org
- www.obesityhelp.com
- www.amos.org
- www.asbs.org
- www.gastricbypass.netfirms.com
- www.VASER.net/consumerinfo.html
- www.soundsurgical.com

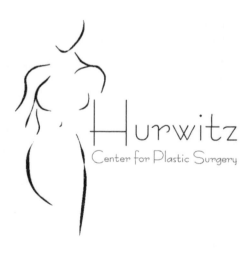

Hurwitz
Center for Plastic Surgery

Index

K

keloids, 147, 148
kidney stones, 35
knee, 1, 11, 12, 23, 55, 60, 74, 78, 79, 81, 83, 87, 90, 91, 99, 100, 103, 104, 154

L

L brachioplasty, 6, 90, 92–96, 112, 119, 124, 163, 164, 169
labia, 83, 89–91, 97–100, 160, 180
laparoscopic technology, 17, 42, 46, 80, 90, 95, 179, 182
laser lipolisis, 68
law of skin laxity, 24, 163
lipoaugmentaton, 3, 103
lipoplasty, 3, 9, 29–31, 53–68, 81, 88, 94, 96, 98, 120, 130, 145, 151, 156, 166, 169, 170, 180, 185
LipoSelection, 31, 67, 90, 97, 100, 130, 166
Lipostabil™, 158
liposuction, 3, 13, 14, 16, 23, 28–31, 55–58, 60–62, 64, 66, 68, 76, 96, 100, 101, 103, 122–124, 130, 131, 139, 145, 151, 160, 166, 172, 180, 181, 184, 185
Lockwood, Ted, 84
lower body lift, 16, 17, 20, 23, 25, 52, 71, 72, 80, 81, 84, 86, 88, 90–97, 99, 101, 103, 112, 114, 115, 119, 145, 155, 163, 169, 170, 181, 184
Lumicel Cell Touch, 157
lung disease, 62
lymphatics, 98, 151, 152
LySonix system, 30, 67

M

Magee Women's Hospital, 1, 4, 7, 24, 65, 68, 142, 164, 168
malabsorption, 41, 43, 44, 140, 183
malnutrition, 140, 167
manual lymphatic drainage, 151
MAO inhibitor, 139
massive weight loss, 6, 16, 17, 22–24, 28, 58, 60, 70, 72, 74, 78, 84, 86, 88, 92, 99, 103, 106, 112, 115, 120, 131, 139, 155, 160, 163, 166, 167, 173, 182
mastopexy, 6, 16, 71, 95, 106, 107, 109, 110, 112–115, 117, 177, 183, 185
medial thighplasty, 6, 16, 23, 71, 89, 90, 99, 103, 115, 170, 184
melatonin, 139
menopause, 71, 100, 153
metabolism, 33, 155, 180
MicroAire®, 68
mons pubis, 78, 79, 81, 82, 86, 88, 98, 160, 183
morbid obesity, 17, 34, 37
Musgrave, Ross, 20

N

narcotics, 63, 137, 142, 165, 181
National Center for Chronic Disease Prevention and Health Promotion, 33
National Health and Nutrition Examination Survey, 32
National Institute of Diabetes and Digestive and Kidney Diseases, 36
neck, 23, 29, 51, 55, 61, 62, 74, 94, 121, 184
necrosis, 29, 60, 119, 136, 183
neurological system, 62
nipple areolar complex, 29, 109, 112, 129, 164, 183, 185
nipple, 28, 29, 56, 71, 89, 94, 106, 109–113, 119, 126, 128, 129, 131, 162, 164, 174, 179, 183, 185
nutrition, 18, 28, 32, 38, 39, 44, 45, 60, 70, 140, 142, 167

swelling, 66, 72, 76, 78, 94, 95, 98, 123, 130, 136, 139, 143, 144, 150, 152, 154, 158, 165, 179, 180
syringe aspirations, 98

T

Tazi, El Hassane, 31, 58
tear drop, 108
tension, 24, 28, 56, 57, 76, 81–85, 89, 91, 93, 97, 98, 113, 117, 118, 143, 160, 161, 163, 179, 182, 184, 185
Tessier, Paul, 21
thalassotherapy, 136, 157
thighplasty, 6, 16, 61, 71, 81, 83, 84, 88–96, 98, 99, 103, 115, 121, 160, 170, 184
Thompson, Tommy, 33
thrombophlebitis, 63, 143, 162, 165
transfusions, 93, 143, 160, 170, 173
transverse scars, 76, 86, 102, 161
TriActive LaserDermology, 157
Tulip® Syringe System, 65
tumescent, 30, 66, 130, 184
type 2 diabetes, 35, 38, 46, 180

U

Ultrashape®, 68
Ultrasonic Assisted Lipoplasty, 30, 31, 59, 66, 67, 94, 96, 120, 130, 157, 166, 185
ultrasound therapy, 152
umbilicoplasty, 185
umbilicus, 78, 80, 81, 83, 88, 97, 98, 100, 101, 109, 113, 160, 162, 166, 181
University of Pittsburgh, 1, 4, 5, 19–21, 34, 46, 48, 72, 75, 76, 86, 142, 164, 175

University of Texas Southwestern, 62
upper body lift, 13, 25, 72, 87–90, 92–96, 106, 112, 114–116, 118–121, 145, 162–164, 169, 170

V

Vaser®, 31, 67, 90, 124, 130, 166, 180, 185, 186
vasoconstrictor, 30, 62, 65, 137, 146, 165, 185
VelaSmooth™ System, 157
VentX™ vented aspiration cannula, 67
vertical banded gastroplasty, 43, 46, 185
vertical inner thighplasty, 81, 83, 95
vertical pattern reduction, 114
vitamin E, 136, 139, 148
vitamins, 45, 136, 138
Vodder, Emil, 152
volume, 18, 24, 30, 31, 56, 59, 62–67, 88, 107, 109–113, 117, 119, 129, 145, 179, 182, 184, 185
vomiting, 45, 46, 140, 143, 167

W

Webster, Jerome, 130
White, William L., 21
Wilson, Carney, 24
Wise pattern mastopexy, 110, 185
wound healing, 25, 28, 76, 143, 145, 146, 177

X

xylocaine, 66, 67, 76, 184
xyphoid, 185

Z

Zook, Elvin, 22
Z-Plasty, 185